Journey to Fitness

Chronicles of a New Triathlete

Linda S. Jassmond Lanfear

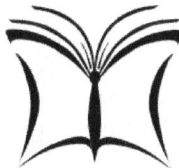

alexemi
PUBLISHING

Exton, Pennsylvania

Please note: This book is intended for informational purposes only and is not to be used as a substitute for professional medical care or treatment. If you suspect you have a medical problem, we urge you to seek competent medical help. Neither the author nor the publisher can be held responsible for any damage, injury, or otherwise resulting from the use of the information in this book.

Mention of any specific company, location, organization, or authority in this book does not imply endorsement by the author or publisher, nor does mention of specific company, location, organization, or authority imply that they endorse the book, its author, or the publisher.

First Edition

Library of Congress Control Number LCCN 2009941624

ISBN 978-0-9815954-3-6

Published by:
Alexemi Publishing
P.O. Box 1266
Exton, PA 19341
www.alexemipublishing.com

Book Cover Design: Jessica Barnak
Back Cover Design: GK Productions, Inc.

Interior Layout: GK Productions, Inc.

Cover Photo: Jessica Barnak, Jessica Barnak Photography

Hair by: Jillian Tuskweth, Jillian Grace Salon

Printed in the U.S.A. 2010

For Jackie, you really are a triathlete!

Acknowledgements

Mom and Dad — thanks for always being there.

GK Productions, Inc. — you are the best at what you do.

Cheryl — I appreciate your expertise.

Kasey — thanks for being a part of this journey.

Contents

Prologue

by Linda S. Jassmond Lanfear

In 2009 I published my first book, *Journey to Fitness — Chronicles of a Working Woman*. It was an inspiring and motivating story about Suzanne, a working mother of three boys and her struggle to find time to work out. Suzanne's initial goal was to feel better in her own skin. There was no mention of weight loss when we started working together and yet she lost 20 pounds during her journey.

Something else happened during Suzanne's transformation that she never saw coming; Suzanne was able to erase 30 years of self-doubt in just one day. Her newfound self-confidence allowed her to achieve many exciting things in all areas of her life!

Journey to Fitness — Chronicles of a New Triathlete is about Jackie, also a working mother. She has a boy and girl and infrequently worked out. I suggested to Jackie that she compete in a triathlon, which would require her to swim, bike and then run. Her answer was classic, "I can't swim. I don't own a bike and I hate to run!"

Another huge obstacle for Jackie was that she refused to swim in a lake, river or ocean. Well, the majority of triathlons are held in, you guessed it, lakes, rivers or oceans. Jackie was a challenge not only from a physical standpoint, but a mental standpoint as well. I had my work cut out for me, but I'm always up for the task.

How was I going to convince Jackie that she could compete in these three sports? If I focused on them one at a time and built up her confidence maybe she would catch the bug...the triathlon bug.

If not, she could possibly sink during the swim and think I was a horrible trainer.

There are lessons to be learned when you take on a new challenge. You change and grow in unexpected ways. Sometimes you realize the people closest to you are not who you thought they were. Read on to follow Jackie on her way to her first possible triathlon…

Every Journey Has A Beginning

When Jackie crossed the finish line, she slumped to the ground. Her hands shook so violently she couldn't hold her water bottle. Even her forehead was shaking. That morning, Jackie had pushed her body further than ever before and she was so proud. It was truly a celebration of determination and accomplishment. She smiled at me with her shaky smile.

> *"I fought with myself a lot this past year while training. I asked myself why I was doing this? Today, I figured it out."*

It was hard to believe that just a year earlier she had told me she couldn't swim, didn't own a bike and hated to run. Now she was a triathlete!

As a personal trainer, people often tell me that they really need to do something to get in shape. Some of them mean it and some of them don't — I think it's just what they expect me to hear. I knew Jackie from teaching fitness classes at the local YMCA. She only attended sporadically, so when she was in class I always made sure to say hello. A lack of "time for themselves" is very common for moms because of children, a significant other, and chores to be done. Sadly, time to work out is typically last on the To Do List. This was the case for Jackie.

Jackie's journey began with a chance meeting. I hadn't seen her for awhile, and then we became reacquainted at a local Business and Professional Women (BPW) networking meeting in July. I had let my previous membership lapse because of my schedule and when I returned years later, Jackie was the organization's president. Small world! She admitted to me that she had been slacking off lately in her workout program, but she was hoping to see me again soon in class. People have the best intentions but don't always follow through with them. A couple of months went by and I didn't see Jackie at the YMCA.

Then in September, I had a chance to talk with Jackie after the monthly BPW meeting. She confessed that she wanted to work out more consistently, so I mentioned working towards a goal like a triathlon.

> She said she always wanted to try one but laughed, "I can't swim. I don't own a bike and I hate to run!"

I assumed it was a dead issue with a statement like that. Imagine my surprise when Jackie showed up in my body sculpting class at the YMCA twice within one week. It was an even bigger surprise to see her in my kickboxing class. Shortly afterward she asked how my mornings looked and if she could schedule a training session with me. She was actually interested in training for a triathlon.

> I asked Jackie when she thought she might like to try a race, and she responded, "I'd like to try one in the spring. I don't want to wait too long before trying one."

I was amazed! There was clearly something inside of her pushing her to do something far beyond what she was currently capable of doing. Jackie thought the first week in October would be a good time to start. We picked October 2nd at 9:00 am to meet. Then something hit me; I would want to bring someone along. Kasey had been a client of mine, then I recruited her to become certified as a personal trainer and work with me. I had helped Kasey and her husband train for triathlons, so she was the perfect person to work with Jackie.

At the beginning of October, before we met for our first session, Jackie told me, "You would be proud of me. Well, I'm proud of myself! This is my second week of cycling at the YMCA first thing in the morning at 5:30 am! I always wonder what I am doing getting up at 5:00 am, but then when I get there, I'm glad I did."

Clients always ask when they should work out. They wonder if one time of day is better than the other. Basically, it all boils down to when they have time. For Jackie, early in the morning seemed best for her. Jackie was off to a great start. The journey to her first triathlon had begun!

She's On Her Way

When Kasey and I arrived at Jackie's house on October 2nd, Jackie said, "What are we doing today?" She was anxious to start training! I told her first we would chat for a bit so I could get her health history and discuss her goals.

Jackie was born in 1973 and has two children, Nathan and Kayla. She thought she was around 5'2". When I asked her weight she hesitated, then said 133 pounds, however admitted she didn't own a scale. "As long as my jeans fit, that's what I want," she explained. This was how Jackie gauged her weight, which was perfectly fine. She felt her weight was fairly consistent.

We went through her medical history. Since high blood pressure is in Jackie's family, she would need to keep an eye on that. Her last physical, two months ago, was good — no physical limitations, no broken bones, no surgeries, no allergies and no medications, including herbs. She didn't smoke and only drank wine occasionally on the weekends. She was very healthy; we would have fun working out with her and really pushing her.

> *When I asked about fitness goals she smiled and said, "I just want to be fit. Look like I'm fit. Feel fit."*

Since the word "fit" can be subjective, I would need more detail on her definition of fit. She did not consider herself a sports player but added, "I'll try anything."

The first red flag was when I asked about her exercise habits. "I don't have a specific day, whenever." She tried to go to the YMCA three times a week and said, "I cram it in at the end of the week if I haven't gone earlier in the week." Jackie had no current plan so I realized this was an area we would have to help her with. *Exercise needed to be a priority.*

I asked Jackie which elements of a triathlon she would enjoy the most. After a very long pause she commented that the running would be the hardest part for her since she hadn't run in so long. "I ran before Nathan was born nine years ago," Jackie stated. Since then, she would think about running and start out, but not last long. Jackie wasn't able to pace herself. She told us,

> *"When I run I don't feel light. I feel weighed down."*

The second red flag was when Jackie said she couldn't run around her neighborhood loop without someone stopping her to talk. Her comment made me realize that exercise for her was more social than serious. To combat this, I suggested she run with her music or when stopped, tell that person she would talk with them after she finished her run.

I then asked if there was anything else she wanted to tell us and she gave it a great deal of thought before responding. It was obvious there was a lot going through Jackie's mind. "I have to get a bike," she finally said. I told her that for a triathlon she would want a road bike and not a mountain bike. Kasey then explained the difference between the thin tires on a road bike and how light the bike is versus the thick tires and heavy frame of a mountain bike. A heavier bike would weigh Jackie down and increase her time. Since triathlons are all about time, a lighter bike would be better.

Kasey asked Jackie how she felt about swimming, and Jackie answered,

> *"Is this crazy, doing a triathlon? When will I go to the pool? What do I know about competitive swimming?"*

Again, it was obvious from Jackie's questions and comments that there was a lot of self-doubt. To help reassure her, Kasey told Jackie she would help her with the swimming portion of the triathlon. Kasey is a strong swimmer and an excellent teacher.

When I asked Jackie about her goals and a time frame, her answer was simple:

1. Lose five pounds by the end of the year
2. Get through a triathlon by spring, maybe April or May

After we discussed her goals I steered the conversation to nutrition and eating. "I think I'm okay. I eat fine, but probably need to cut back," Jackie said then continued, "I'm not a big dessert person and I don't eat chips. If I don't have it in front of me I'm fine." It was a great statement and the reason why I recommended Jackie not bring tempting food into the house. If it's not there, she won't look for it. Another topic was hydration and Jackie told me she drinks plenty of water, which is very important.

After covering the basics, we moved on to her training. To help with her lack of weekly planning, she got her calendar and we started to fill it in. Monday she did a 45-minute beginner cycling class. Tuesday was open. Wednesday was also open and she said she could cycle that morning. Thursday and Friday were open. We discussed working out with the family but she said, "It's easier to exercise when I'm on my own." The new plan was to schedule exercise into Jackie's week and leave Saturday and Sunday for family activities. The goal with the plan was to make exercise a priority by scheduling it into her day.

Then she said the magic phrase, which was precisely what I wanted to hear,

"Once it's scheduled, whatever it is, I'll do it."

Kasey explained the importance of cross training, which is exactly what a triathlon is. In addition to cycling, we would help Jackie add other activities, such as running and swimming, to her schedule. Next week Jackie and Kasey agreed to swim together at the YMCA. Kasey explained that swimming a quarter mile, which is what a Sprint Triathlon typically is, would be 18 laps in the pool. We talked about breathing on both sides in case Jackie had a bunch of swimmers on her right side, she could turn to the left. When they go to the pool, Kasey explained they would not push off the wall because Jackie would not be pushing off a wall in a triathlon.

"I actually can't wait to swim!" Jackie said. This was a good sign because she was not a strong swimmer. There was a question about where she'd swim in an actual triathlon and we explained it would typically be in the ocean, a pond, or a lake. Another red flag surfaced — Jackie has a fear of snakes, so swimming someplace other than in a pool was a major concern for her. Kasey and I reassured Jackie that neither one of us had ever seen a snake during a triathlon.

And the run? I told Jackie we would start today. "Oh! I'm worried about running," Jackie said. We headed outside into the sunny 65-degree weather. I was hoping to ride Jackie's husband's bike so I could watch her gait but the tire was off it. It worked out alright though, because Kasey would keep an eye on Jackie and would let me know if she had any concerns.

My goal, I told Jackie, was for her to run around her neighborhood loop without walking, even if she had to do a slow jog. I started my watch and off they went. As they were coming up the hill, I could see them talking — obviously the pace was okay. My watch read 6:50 minutes.

> *"Oh my gosh. I never ran so far before!" Jackie*
> *was excited so I high-fived then hugged her.*

Kasey explained how they started out too fast and she had to slow them down. She felt it should take Jackie around 7:30 to run around the loop, not 6:50 like they just did. Jackie did have to walk for a few steps and Kasey felt it was because of the quick pace. It was almost a sprint so Jackie now knew to slow it down.

Jackie said, "I'm heavier in the butt and thighs." I explained that losing the weight and doing these three different activities along with lifting weights would slim her down. When I asked how she felt, Jackie said she was achy in her back, right above her butt. I told her to keep an eye on this and as long as she feels okay 24 or 48 hours from now, she could run again. Jackie commented about feeling achy in her shoulders and Kasey suggested that Jackie relax a little more while running. Kasey also recommended running two times a week for 30 minutes; one loop could be a walk then run. The minimum Kasey wanted was 15-20 minutes with a goal of 30 minutes. Jackie's first running plan was now in place.

I told Jackie I wanted her to keep a food journal for a week, which would include liquids and exercise. I would give her my journal tablet that evening when I saw her at the BPW meeting. Jackie wanted accountability and asked about our procedures to keep in touch. I explained that when we see clients weekly, they could email as often as they like. If we're seeing clients every other week or once a month, we'll answer quick email questions when we get them, but will go into detail the next time we meet. Having said this, we agreed that Jackie would swim with Kasey the next week and then the three of us would meet again in two weeks.

When Kasey left I explained to Jackie how our meeting was confidential and anything she wanted to tell people about the triathlon was up to her. Jackie voiced concern about telling others, fearing they might have negative comments. She decided to tell them about three months prior to her race. I added that she would also be stronger mentally at that point to handle their comments if they did say anything negative. She also decided to wait and tell her husband Todd about the triathlon around that same time. "There might be negative comments from him too," she frowned.

Her parting thoughts were about swimming in open water. Obviously this was bothering her.

> *"I was serious about the water, what's in it? I have a fear of what's in it. When the kids try to show me frogs, they make me nauseous and squeamish."* I reassured her she'd be okay.

It was a good first meeting and I left a smiling Jackie in her driveway. She was on her way to her first triathlon.

That evening at the BPW meeting, Jackie was telling the group "I'm not an organized person." This comment was important to hear. Jackie will become an organized person if she makes exercise a priority, scheduled into her day.

It surprised me to hear Jackie mention at least three different times over the course of the evening about her running and that I had helped her. She seemed genuinely proud. The group was teasing that I probably used a whip on her — I joked, "No whip, just a bullhorn." It was Jackie's choice to say she ran that day and she told them she felt really good. She hadn't gone public yet about the triathlon, but had told others she was running.

Over the next couple of days, Jackie and Kasey went back and forth by email to set up a date and time to swim. They decided on an early-morning swim at 5:00 am. Jackie explained,

> *"I'm not usually up at that time, but I think if I change the routine, I can get more exercise in since it works around the kids."*

It was so encouraging how Jackie was willing to try something new. She seemed excited about exercising at an early hour of the morning and about the possibility of being able to work around her children.

Kasey told me about a free adult masters swim class at the YMCA. She said the description sounded perfect for Jackie and that she might try it as well. Since the YMCA does not allow outside trainers in to train, there would be no charge for Kasey to help get Jackie acclimated to the pool environment. Kasey said she would fill Jackie in on the swim class when she saw her.

It was then that I had a great idea to pass by Kasey. I asked her what she thought about us chronicling Jackie's journey to a triathlon for my second book. This opportunity was too good to pass up. It could be so motivational to document Jackie's journey from the beginning. I asked Kasey not to mention this to Jackie yet, when the time was right we would tell her.

Just as with Suzanne from my first book, everything would be confidential and when Jackie completed her triathlon, she would have the opportunity to read and edit the book. Kasey loved the idea! Now, it was up to Jackie. I felt confident that Jackie would follow through with a triathlon, especially because she had both of us backing her. We were on our way!

Jackie Gets Her Toes Wet

Kasey and Jackie met for their first swim on October 12th at 5:30 am. I wish I could have been there. Seeing the progress from a client's first time in a pool through to a triathlon is exciting. Actually, it's exciting to see anyone do anything for the first time and then watch them progress.

Kasey filled me in on the morning and told me that she thought it went well. Some of the highlights included swimming a total of 18 laps, one lap at a time. Only once did Kasey push Jackie to swim two in a row. Jackie never learned how to do a proper freestyle so she didn't put her head in the water. This was where they focused; practicing a lot of breathing and working on keeping Jackie's head down. Kasey felt there was a huge improvement during the hour.

> *Jackie noted, "This morning it wasn't hard to*
> *get up to meet Kasey at the YMCA. I was kind*
> *of excited and nervous to get there. I got into*
> *the water and Kasey asked me to swim just like*
> *I would normally so she could see what I knew*
> *already. She also told me we would be doing*
> *at least 15 laps today. Cool, I thought. I can do*
> *that. So I did my sidestroke and my freestyle*
> *with my head out of the water up and then back.*
> *When I finished, I couldn't breathe! I was out of*
> *breath after only two laps!"*

In total they completed Kasey's goal of 18 laps, which was a quarter mile. For several of the laps Kasey put a buoy in between Jackie's legs to just practice her arms and breathing. Two laps were using the kick board to practice kicking. Jackie thought this was extremely difficult and couldn't make it across the pool without stopping. Kasey observed that Jackie was using her right leg to kick much harder than her left so they worked on that as well. Kasey timed a few laps and the average was 40-45 seconds each. At the end, she asked Jackie to do one lap as fast as she could and she did it in 25 seconds! There was a big difference when Jackie kept her head down and in the water.

Overall, Jackie was very pleased with her performance and was excited about swimming. However, she did feel it was a lot harder than she imagined it would be and she had to rest between most laps to regulate her breathing. Kasey suggested Jackie look into the masters swim classes offered there at the YMCA to enhance endurance, stroke mechanics and work on race training. The coaches would tailor the workouts from the beginner level to the more experienced swimmer. Jackie agreed to look into it.

Later in the day Jackie was very tired. I explained to her that like anything new, it would be hard for awhile, but then she would be okay. We agreed to meet again on October 23rd. Finding a date which worked for both Jackie and Kasey was a challenge because of their children's schedules. Not having children myself, I am always amazed at how moms get things done. They constantly have to juggle schedules. We agreed to meet at Jackie's home again for our next session. For the following week or so, Jackie would be on her own to work out.

Training Solo

The next week Jackie signed up for the masters swim class as Kasey suggested. Even though the class wouldn't be starting until the beginning of November, it was a very positive sign; we were able to get Jackie interested enough and confident enough to sign up for the class. I could almost guarantee she would not have signed up if Kasey hadn't worked with her in the pool.

Kasey and I made plans for our next session with Jackie. We would talk about how things were going and then walk/run for at least 30 minutes, followed by some strengthening exercises. Since we hadn't seen Jackie's food journal yet, we would need to take the time to go through it. I had only given Jackie a week's worth of food journal sheets, so we would need to assess if this would be something we wanted Jackie to keep on a regular basis.

For the strength training exercises, I asked Kasey to write down each exercise, what weight, and approximately how many reps for Jackie to start with. We would get right into the exercises with me there, and after I left Kasey would review the food journal. The plan was now in place.

The Monday after their first swim, I taught my usual classes at the YMCA. When I was leaving the building I walked past the "testosterone" room (we call it that because all the very muscular guys congregate in there). I saw Jackie working out on a piece of equipment. I stopped in to say hi. She told me she had slept in that morning and missed her cycling class, so she was working out on the weight machines instead. She mentioned that her right shoulder hurt. I recommended she take it easy with the weight machines and not push it. Jackie added that when she cycles her arms and shoulders were getting tingly. I suggested she put less pressure on the handle bars — sometimes people push down so hard into the handle bars and there's no need. Jackie said she could feel her shoulder when she runs too and thinks she's hunching.

I contacted Kasey with the Jackie update so she would be prepared for our next session. Our once-sedentary client was now swimming, biking, running and lifting weights! We would need to pace her. I don't mind clients saying they're achy for a day or two, but when the pain doesn't go away, it needs to be addressed.

Jackie continued to work on her swimming on her own. She worked on getting her head in the water to get more comfortable. She would jump in the pool and stand there for 5-10 minutes before working up the courage to swim off. Then after getting used to the water with her head down, she worked on breathing in the water and taking a breath on every third stroke. This was a challenge for Jackie and it took her several pool visits to find a rhythm.

> *"Swimming was kind of frustrating I have to say. I hated it at times. I thought running would be my number one dislike, but it turned out to be the swimming. I thought I was just going to jump in the water and start swimming like an Olympian. I was wrong!"*

Every time Jackie went to the pool she would get advice from the people swimming around her and was able to pick up some helpful pointers. She started using the buoys that fit between her knees just to get her stroke down and improve her breathing. She even swam a few times with friends. Then Jackie joined a triathlon class at the YMCA, which met weekly, and swam with other people who were also learning.

Consistency in the water is the key to mastering the swim. Most importantly, she learned not to give up and go home. Jackie laughed when she told me, "I figured I couldn't get much worse than I already was, so there only had to be room for improvement, right?" Jackie was really taking her solo workouts seriously.

One day I stopped by an open house at a local business and much to my surprise, Jackie was there. She is a cooking consultant and had provided a lot of the food, which was delicious. Jackie looked great! She always dressed nicely, but looked particularly good that evening. I often notice that something happens to my clients when they start working out and begin to understand what we are trying to teach them. They smile more and appear more confident.

Jackie told me she already felt a few pounds lighter. She talked about how much she liked the track at the YMCA. When she went for a run outside, she felt heavy, like she was pulling a cart. She also told me she had played tennis with a friend recently after not playing for eight years. Tennis was something new and different to do, so she and her friend agreed they would continue to play when they could.

She brought up the triathlon a few times and said she would like to be able to listen to music during the race. I explained that she wouldn't need it because she would be so focused. Jackie mentioned a friend of hers who had completed a few triathlons and was inquiring about Jackie's so she could do it with her.

> *Jackie, being unsure of herself, decided to do her first triathlon alone and I agreed with her.*

There was no mention at all about her shoulder pain so I hoped it was on the mend.

Pounding The Pavement

Jackie, Kasey and I met for our second group meeting on October 23rd. When I drove into Jackie's neighborhood, I realized I needed to clock the mileage for the loop that she and Kasey ran the last time. When I got to the house, Kasey was there. She also had clocked the mileage and it was .6 miles, a little more than a half mile.

It was 8:30 am and we didn't go into the living room this time, we stood in the hall and chatted. Her husband Todd was upstairs getting ready for work. Our conversation was generic since Jackie had only told him bits and pieces about working with us, but not about the triathlon.

We would definitely need to keep an eye on Jackie's right shoulder, since she said it was still bothering her. Jackie mentioned that a few days before our meeting, she swam 18 laps just like she and Kasey had done, minus the flotation device. She said she's "sore" even when she first gets out of bed. We had taken an inconsistent exerciser and now have her working out on a regular basis. We needed to help pace her.

Jackie ran twice earlier in the week but didn't time it and asked us not to talk about time with her husband around. He was so competitive that he might not realize she would prefer a pat on the back rather than making everything a competition.

Jackie got up early to cycle one morning, then went home and slept for 15 minutes before the kids got up. What did she give up for triathlons? She gave up nothing, except a little of her personal time.

*In fact she now felt this **was** her personal time —
going out to exercise was a way to release stress
and to focus. It was also a way to get away from
all the hustle and bustle of real life. She actually
found she was becoming more organized with
her life; she was making every minute count.
Her dedication was admirable.*

She could now admit she liked having exercise scheduled because it ensured that she would do it. We talked about that on our first visit and I suggested she schedule exercise into her calendar. Because she put it on the calendar she had been successful at attending classes, running and swimming. *Planning does work.*

We stretched as we talked. Jackie said her right shoulder hurt even just stretching. I was really getting concerned about it.

We went outside and were treated to a gorgeous late October day; 70 degrees, a bit breezy and overcast, but the sun was peeking through. Kasey wanted to set a slow pace and go around the loop two times without stopping. Jackie decided not to take her music player. Excellent, I thought, because it would give them a chance to talk and bond. I was going to bring my bike, but decided against it. This was a time for Jackie to really trust Kasey, which was important. I watched and was the timekeeper.

As they came up the hill, I pumped my arms and Kasey said, "One down." Their time was 7:23 for .6 miles, which was a good slow pace. As they ran up the hill the second lap, I pumped my arms again. I could hear them talking and laughing. The time was 15:10 and it was the first time Jackie had run nonstop for two laps. Jackie needed water so I ran along side them and gave her the water bottle. She commented that it was hard to run and swallow, then handed the bottle back to me. During a race, she would appreciate the water and will have no problem exercising and swallowing water.

They came up the hill for the third lap, and they were still talking; an indication that they were keeping a steady pace. It had been 23 minutes and Todd was now outside so I flashed them the number two and number three with my fingers. I didn't mention time in front of Todd as Jackie requested. Kasey said, "Let's go to the end of the hill and see how you feel." I watched them continue to run past the bottom of the hill.

Todd asked, "Are you working her hard? I think she said she's trying to get up to five miles. I'm not a runner — never liked it. How far is it around here?" I responded that yes, we were working her hard and she was doing a great job. I didn't say anything about the triathlon, but told him it's .6 miles around the loop. As Todd left I spotted the girls laughing and talking. I pumped my arms with excitement because so far it was 28 minutes of nonstop running. Kasey had Jackie drop both arms straight down to relax her shoulders.

Jackie was holding her left arm a bit higher than her right when she came up the hill. Jackie said, "Oh my gosh," realizing she had run nonstop for 2.4 miles — four loops in 31 minutes. We were all excited and walked to the bottom of the hill then back up again. Jackie had run non-stop!

> *"I remember in high school when we used to have to run around the track four times in gym class," Jackie recalled and added, "I may have been one of the only girls who got sick to my stomach, felt faint, and had horrible side pains! I would have to ask the gym teacher if I could sit down before I fell over, but it felt great to run today. I think I'm getting over my fear of running and might even tell some people my plans. Not Todd yet though, I still have a lot of work to do before I take that leap!"*

Kasey told me that Jackie talked the entire time they ran. "I feel tightness in my chest," Jackie said, like she had a cold. Most likely it was just part of getting her lungs conditioned but we would certainly keep an eye on it. Jackie said she would buy a watch and explained she was buying one thing at a time. She also commented she needed new sneakers. I liked the way she was buying things gradually and hoped she viewed these purchases as investments in her training. She was worth it.

They continued to stretch outside while we chatted. As I was leaving Jackie said, "I actually feel good! We'll see how I feel tomorrow." When I left they went inside to work out with weights.

I had to leave to meet with my next client. As I was driving away I thought about how much I would have liked to be with them to hear the conversation of the run and the excitement of Jackie having just run nonstop for 31 minutes.

Later I caught up with Kasey who told me what a good job Jackie had done with the weights. Jackie's food journal looked fine; she had healthy eating habits. Jackie was not interested in continuing with the journal for now. Her eating did not appear out of line, so that was okay with me. Sometimes a trainer needs to decide for the client, but Jackie only wanted to lose five pounds by the end of the year, so the journal wasn't as critical. If she started to gain on the scale or her clothes felt tight, we might need her to keep a journal.

It had been a productive day of training!

I Think I Can, I Think I Can

The day after our second group meeting Jackie felt great. Her legs weren't sore from the run, but her shoulder was still bothering her. Jackie agreed to stay cognizant of how her shoulder felt over the next few days. The idea was to try and determine what was irritating the shoulder so she could cut back on any exercises bothering it.

Jackie was running again the following day; this time inside at the YMCA because it was raining. She ran for 30 minutes, but lost track of the number of laps. She felt that she actually ran a longer distance than she had run with Kasey, since running on a track with no hills was easier. Her shoulder was not too bad and she was starting to think it was the swimming causing the irritation. She hoped if she swam once a week her shoulder would eventually improve.

A few days later, my husband and I were grocery shopping when we saw Jackie with her two children.

> *She was so excited to tell me that she was*
> *recently able to stroke three times then take a*
> *breath when swimming. Jackie mimicked the*
> *stroke motions. And yes, she was breathing on*
> *both sides.*

She said she liked to go to the pool when she thought no one would be there. But, as luck would have it, her neighbor showed up one day and swam in the lane next to her.

In the grocery store Jackie looked so cute and had such a wonderful smile on her face. You could tell that she was feeling better about what she was trying to accomplish. I was concerned however, with her comment about wanting to swim when no one was around. To me, that meant she was still apprehensive about swimming. Someday such comments would be gone and she would like people swimming next to her. It was the progression of confidence and something I thoroughly enjoy hearing and seeing.

The Word Was Out

At a November Business Card Exchange, Jackie and I pulled into the parking lot at the same time and we walked in together. She looked great, smiling and happy. We chatted while setting up and she was proud to say she had jogged three miles that week. When I asked how her shoulder was doing, she said she couldn't do a headstand with her daughter but she could do a push up, though with some pain. "It's from swimming," she said motioning to her shoulder. She could be right and should see a doctor.

Jackie still preferred going to the YMCA to swim when no one was there, but now when she runs into someone she knows she doesn't let it stop her from swimming. "I can't wait to go back!" she blurted. She would soon get the chance when the masters swim class at the YMCA started that Saturday.

As we were meeting and greeting people at the card exchange, I heard Jackie talking about her triathlon. She mentioned she didn't want to wait until August to do a triathlon; she wanted one in April.

> Jackie then declared, "I'm going to do both an
> April triathlon and then another in August,"
> which really surprised me.

The word was out that Jackie will participate in a triathlon and she was the one spreading the word! One woman told Jackie she likes running alone, but Jackie told her she prefers running with someone. They continued to talk about running and Jackie told her and others about how she had been searching the internet looking for triathlons.

*Jackie laughed when she told us she went to a
5:30 am cycling class, but was shocked that it
was full by the time she got there. "Who goes
to a 5:30 am class?" she said. "I guess a lot of
people do! I did some weights instead and the
rowing machine for 20 minutes."*

There was a time when she may have just gone home if faced with
a full class, but not the new and improved, fitness-minded Jackie!

She was on the right track and would need to remain focused to
meet her goals. I would have preferred to see her more frequently,
but sometimes it just doesn't work out that way. Clients often think
a detailed email to their trainer is enough so they put off seeing
us for another week. I like to see them in person. However, since
we were in the building phase with a highly motivated Jackie, I
wasn't worried about the sporadic visits. Connecting with her at
networking events gave me the opportunity to check in with her
from time to time. With all the work Jackie was doing, I knew she
would be okay for the race.

Jackie invited me to a home show the following week. I try to
attend one event per client whenever I can to see them in a non-
fitness environment. On this occasion I'm glad I went because
another client was there, as was Kasey.

Jackie looked attractive in a black and white ruffled blouse. The
home show was for a popular line of clothing and Jackie was
asked to model several different outfits. She looked stunning in
each one, especially the black sheer dress. Everyone commented
that Jackie would look good in anything and I agreed. Jackie is
blessed with a nice height and a nice figure. Her variety of exercises was toning and slimming her body. She wanted to lose five
pounds and was on her way to achieving her goal.

She was modeling clothes in front of a group of us and the clothing rep was having Jackie turn around so we could see how the
clothes made Jackie's butt look. I wondered if she would have
been comfortable modeling clothes prior to working with us. I
wasn't so sure. I could sense her increased self confidence. Jackie
seemed happy. This is part of what we do — we help people build
confidence.

At the November BPW meeting Jackie told us about a tri-suit she bought off the internet. It sounded like a unitard with a zippered front, padded butt for the bike, and was about shorts length. Jackie said the suit would be mailed to her in a few days. I wished I could be there when she opened the box — reality would hit her that she was really going to be competing in a triathlon!

Jackie told me about a friend, who competes in triathlons. She asked Jackie to come south to do one with her on December 8th. The friend lives near the ocean, so it would be an ocean swim. Jackie felt it would be too soon because she would be afraid of the swim. I agreed, it would be too early in her training for Jackie to compete, especially if the swim was longer than a quarter mile.

Jackie talked about being able to walk her bike or walk during the run if she needed to. However she couldn't walk in the ocean. She wanted time to practice techniques to take breaks in the water. I mentioned she might try sidestroke or breaststroke, things she could do if she got too tired and needed to catch her breath.

The first week in December Jackie had her shoulder examined. The doctor felt that she had overworked her rotator cuff causing bursitis. He gave her some exercises to do and agreed that the swimming likely caused it. She cut back on her workouts for awhile and planned to swim just a little at a time. "I probably won't push it too much," she told me but seemed frustrated.

> *"Swimming is my biggest challenge! Maybe we can meet up and swim soon. I can work on the other things myself but I really need help with the swimming."*

Kasey and I were concerned about Jackie's shoulder. Sometimes new clients get so excited when they start a fitness program they have a tendency to overdo it. We set limits for clients, knowing this can happen. Unfortunately much of Jackie's training had been done on her own, and we couldn't officially work with Jackie in the pool since it was against YMCA rules. Kasey couldn't see her competing in a triathlon until she significantly improved her stroke, but swimming might aggravate the bursitis in her shoulder.

When I walked into the BPW December meeting, Jackie looked so pretty. That woman could wear anything and look good! Within minutes of taking my seat Jackie came over to talk to me about her shoulder. I asked how often and how long she was swimming. She was swimming on her own about once a week for an hour at a time. I suggested she swim twice a week for 20 minutes. I also emphasized the importance of listening to her doctor and doing the exercises he gave her.

Jackie then said a friend, who is a swimmer, told her she was reaching too much with her stroke. The friend told Jackie to almost scratch her face with her thumb and Jackie said she would try it. I didn't want to say this in front of the group, but I become concerned when someone other than a professional gives advice to a client and then the client follows it. There is a chance for misinterpretation and I wouldn't want any client getting hurt.

What would happen if Jackie misunderstood her friend and tried something that injured her shoulder? Ugh! This is why I like to see clients weekly to keep track of training and help eliminate such problems. I always start my clients out slow and exercise on the side of caution.

After the December BPW meeting, almost a month went by without hearing from Jackie. When we finally caught up, Jackie told me the holidays went fine and although she did not exercise as much as usual, she didn't really overeat and was able to maintain her weight. She had a cortisone injection in her shoulder which took away some of her pain, but it was still bothering her. The doctor said that would happen — she would have some pain after the shot, but eventually the pain would go away.

She planned to start swimming again gradually, only a few laps at a time. Jackie was continuing to run indoors on the track or treadmill and had been taking yoga and Pilates classes. She wanted to start to bike outside, but didn't get a bike for Christmas as she was hoping. I offered to bring some bikes over that we could use and we agreed to set up another group session soon. I was glad to hear she was listening to her body and not pushing her shoulder too hard.

Group Support

At the January BPW meeting Jackie showed me the new sneakers she was given for Christmas. She now spoke openly about
triathlons. I was the guest speaker for the evening and as Jackie
introduced me, she told the group that I work with novices as well
as those clients training for a triathlon. I asked Jackie if she would
like to share with the group about her triathlon.

We hadn't rehearsed it, so Jackie spoke off the top of her head.
She told the group she had talked to me after a BPW meeting one
evening and I suggested she do a triathlon. She explained that at
the time, she couldn't swim, didn't own a bike and she hated to
run.

> *"I now run three and a half miles, I bike and I*
> *swim," she stated proudly.*

She also told them about the unitard she bought for triathlons and
talked about her plans to compete in a triathlon in the spring.

We chatted a few minutes about it and we all agreed we should
support Jackie, especially by going to her first race. Someone
even suggested we get BPW t-shirts made up with Jackie's name
on them. How cool would that be — a group of women wearing
"Go Jackie" shirts and cheering for her. I was ecstatic for Jackie;
a woman without the skills or equipment needed to do a triathlon,
yet she still had the desire. I really believe all we need is desire
and we can do it. In this respect Jackie excelled!

Our game plan changed shortly after the BPW meeting, because
Jackie discovered an upcoming indoor triathlon on March 2nd.
The event would include a 10-minute swim in the pool, 30 min-
utes on a stationary bike, and then 20 minutes on a treadmill. The

results would be based on the distance achieved within each time frame. Jackie felt this would be a good way to start out and eliminate some of her anxiety about competing in a bigger outdoor triathlon.

An indoor triathlon may actually be good as a pre-cursor to a more rigorous outdoor event. Jackie would have to be the best judge of her shoulder. Ten minutes in a pool wouldn't be too bad if she was able to use the wall to push off. If she was in her own lane (assuming they had staggered starts) she would have the luxury of going as slowly as she needed and do the sidestroke to get through it.

Kasey and I agreed that Jackie should sign up for it. If Jackie needed help her with transitions, we could work with her. It would be important to train doing multiple exercises back to back (they are called bricks) i.e., bike/run or swim/bike. Jackie's body would get the feel for transitioning between the different events.

I told Cheryl, my Virtual Author's Assistant, about the indoor triathlon and mentioned that Jackie's story could possibly be book number two. "So cool — you're right about Jackie being highly motivated!" Cheryl responded. It was true, what made Jackie think she could compete in a triathlon? We gave her the basic skills and encouraged her to go for it — amazingly — Jackie was planning to go through with it!

Pressing The Enter Button

I nearly fell out of my chair when Jackie announced excitedly on the morning of January 23rd,

> *"OK, I signed up for it!! I can't believe I just did it!" She went on to say, "I'm really nervous! The race is March 2nd and I signed up for the 10:40 am heat. It was so hard to press the enter button to sign up! Talking about doing the triathlon is one thing, but doing it is another story. NOW it seems real!"*

I was thrilled for Jackie, but a little disappointed for me. It turns out that my mom's 75th birthday was March 1st and our entire family would be with her in Florida to celebrate. My dad was having a party for her. This race would be huge for Jackie, absolutely amazing, and I wanted to be there. Do I go to Florida then take a late flight home that evening?

What happens if Jackie ends up not going to the triathlon? There was the possibility she or her children could get sick or something else could come up to prevent her from participating. I thought of Kasey going in my place to watch the race, but then Cheryl came to mind because she had been working with me on my first book and was aware that Jackie might be book number two. Darn — two awesome things happening on the same weekend.

Participating in a race is so exhilarating. I love to see my clients cross the finish line; they're so excited! It lets them know what they can achieve — then their self-confidence soars. Because of the multiple parts of a triathlon — swimming, biking, and running — it's different from a regular race. After riding a certain amount of miles it is a difficult transition for the body, particularly the legs, to get off the bike then start to run. I've watched clients finish a 5 or 10K race, but there is something special about a triathlon; there is so much more emotion.

I couldn't believe I was going to miss Jackie's first triathlon. My other thought was what happens if the BPW gang is all there? It would be an amazing thing to witness, everyone jumping up and down. I was torn, but I knew I wanted to be with my mom to support her at her big event.

That afternoon I contacted Cheryl and asked her if attending triathlons was anywhere in her job description. I filled her in on the situation, how she could take pictures and write about the event if she were there. I emphasized that the first race would be special because of the ultimate excitement for the client, especially when they cross the finish line.

Cheryl didn't think she really had a formal job description in her work with me, but if she did, attending a triathlon to help with a future book would certainly fit in. She would be there to be my eyes and ears.

Now that Jackie had a firm race date, she would have a concrete goal to work towards. Kasey and I offered to help Jackie train. It would be interesting to see if Jackie felt she needed our help or if she wanted to try to figure this out on her own.

As I thought about Jackie's triathlon, I considered sending Cheryl all that I had written about Jackie so she would have background on everything we had done. Or maybe I should let Cheryl meet Jackie for the first time without any background or history. I also thought of showing Cheryl pictures of a triathlon so she would know what to expect. Sure this one would be indoors, but the participants would still swim, bike and run.

I was thinking about Jackie; she would be excited and nervous, but I also knew she would do well. I could imagine her face when she finished and it would have a big smile on it. I always try to remind clients that when they have their first race they should have fun. When Kasey competed in a triathlon she told me she had a few goals in mind in terms of time and not being the last one to cross the finish line. Goals are good but they need to be realistic. I would have to remind Jackie of this.

A few days passed and I didn't hear from Jackie so I was hoping to catch up with her at our February BPW meeting. When I arrived at the meeting Jackie exclaimed to me that she *liked* swimming and felt Kasey would be impressed with her progress. Kasey first saw Jackie when she didn't know how to swim — it was very different now.

I asked Jackie about her shoulder and she said it still hurt, even after the cortisone shot. Jackie asked what she should do about it and I told her she needed to talk with her doctor and to rest it as much as possible. Of course she didn't like the idea, but she really needed to give her shoulder a chance to heal.

It was a small BPW meeting, half the group we had the previous month. I was waiting to hear if Jackie would announce her triathlon, but she didn't. Not a word about her March date. Interesting.

The evening presentation was on dentistry and Jackie told us she had braces when she was a kid. She made us laugh when she talked about wearing her headgear to school. Depending on your age you might remember it, a silver bar that hooks into the braces with an elastic strap holding it around your head. Jackie said she was told to wear it eight hours a day. Most people would wear it at night, but she wore it to school even though she felt uncomfortable with what people thought. I felt that statement really summed up Jackie's personality:

> *"Even when I was younger I was afraid of*
> *what people thought of me," she said, "but I*
> *was willing to take chances." It is interesting,*
> *though, she was not willing to tell Todd or others*
> *close to her, about her triathlon. Their opinions*
> *meant a lot to her.*

After the meeting a few of us hung around to talk. Jackie mentioned that even though she was working out she was not losing much weight. I asked about her clothes and she admitted they did fit better since she started to exercise. I pointed out that this was a good sign for her; fitness is not all about pounds or a number on the scale. I suggested she keep an eye on her food portions and to continue drinking plenty of water. I didn't want to give her too much information — I wanted to sit down to talk with her.

Jackie updated me, via email, on her training. She had been working to build her endurance while swimming, but her biggest concerns about the upcoming race were with the logistics of the race itself. "I have never done a triathlon before," she said, "and what I need help with is what to expect even though this one will be indoors. What do I wear? How do I go from swimming to biking? Where do my sneakers go? I know these all sound like simple questions, but I have no idea of how that works. What I wouldn't mind is a practice run of the transitions of the indoor triathlon. I go from 10 minutes of swimming, to 30 minutes of biking, to 20 minutes of running," Jackie added.

Those were great questions which we would have already reviewed if we had been seeing each other on a regular basis. Now we would need to backtrack to fill in the gaps. With any race, preparation and practice are essential; this is especially true for a triathlon. Transitions are important because time can be lost in them. Every second of a triathlon counts. There's a certain way to pile your clothes, what items to have there, what clothes to wear, what food to have, water, and so on. I suggested to Jackie we set up a time to meet to answer all of her questions and address her concerns.

From what Kasey had read she was under the impression the participants would be allotted 10 minutes to change from swimming to bike clothes for this special event. Wow, if this were so, it would be a gift. Typically, a participant will only take a minute or two. With this being an indoor race, I assumed they wanted participants to be totally dry so they don't drip all over the bikes and treadmills.

My one regret was not being able to train Jackie more for this event but it was her choice. I was psyched that this woman who didn't know how to swim, didn't own a bike and hated to run was actually competing in a triathlon. Talk about stepping outside of your comfort zone! Jackie agreed to meet with Kasey and me on

February 27th to go over the logistics of the race to help prepare her.

A couple days later, I had an idea. What if Kasey did a practice triathlon with Jackie which would give her some competition? I passed this by Kasey and asked how she would feel about actually doing the swim, bike and run with Jackie on the 27th. She said she would — although she hoped she could keep up with Jackie since she hadn't been swimming in a long time.

I was glad that Kasey agreed — it would work out well. Preparation is key. We tell this to our clients all the time, but it's ultimately their decision on what to do. If Jackie hadn't practiced transitions (moving from the swim, to the bike, to the run) she would be at a disadvantage.

I filled Jackie in and told her that whatever she had been wearing for training is what she should bring for the practice triathlon. If she was comfortable with it, wear it. If she wanted to wear something different, she should wear it for the next two weeks. I emphasized the importance of being comfortable with the clothes she's wearing the entire time she's doing each part of this race. Again, this is where planning comes in. It doesn't matter if it's for a race or packing your lunch — so you don't get stuck eating at a fast food restaurant — *planning is key.*

Kasey contacted Jackie to highlight some things she should bring for the practice triathlon. The list included swim suit, goggles, swim cap or hair tie, towel, sneakers, under garments for bike/run, shorts, t-shirt, good socks, water and/or sports drink and music player.

Kasey and I had very different approaches because I wanted to see what Jackie would bring, but Kasey spelled it out for her. When I first work with clients I let them think through the process and get a list in their heads of what they'll need. This helps them plan. Jackie was unique, however, because she had been training on her own. Since Kasey gave her a list, Jackie was set. In this case, I think it helped ease Jackie's mind.

It was my idea to do the practice triathlon, but I was a little apprehensive since we would be swimming, biking and running so close to her actual triathlon Typically, I would not do this because it was just way too close. I knew I would have to keep a close eye on Jackie to make sure she was okay and didn't endanger herself for the actual race.

I decided to send Cheryl everything I had written so she could get to know a little bit more about Jackie. I explained that I hadn't revealed anything to Jackie yet about the possibility of writing a book. I wanted to capture her raw emotions. I didn't think Jackie knew much about Suzanne's book at the time so I wanted to keep her in the dark for now. I also reminded Cheryl to take notes during the triathlon. Anything she saw, write it down. Times, what time did Jackie start? How long did it take Jackie to change? Was Jackie's family there? Were they supportive? Cheryl would fill me in.

We decided to tell Jackie that I was sending Cheryl to take some photos for me to document the race in case we wanted to use them later on my website. This way, Jackie wouldn't think a stranger was taking photos of her.

When I told Jackie that Cheryl would be there, she responded, "Great! I did want pictures, but I wasn't planning on anyone going with me!"

This struck me as odd so I asked Cheryl to observe Jackie closely at the race. What I wanted to know is why wasn't Jackie planning on having anyone go with her? There's psychology with my job. Was she embarrassed? Was she afraid she wouldn't be able to do the triathlon? Did she want to do this alone to prove she could? The members of the BPW had said they wanted to support Jackie at her triathlon, but I now realized she hadn't told anyone about this race. In order to motivate someone it helps me to understand where their mind is.

Cheryl was glad she would be able to be there to document the event and cheer for Jackie. I was equally excited, and I knew Cheryl would thoroughly enjoy it. The thrill of finishing a race and watching someone finish a race is indescribable. I think the pictures Cheryl takes will capture the excitement.

The day before we planned to meet for the practice triathlon, I checked my email one last time before going to bed and I'm glad I did. It was around 10:00 pm and Jackie had sent a message to both Kasey and me. It read,

"Just so you know — and so you can tell me what you think I should do — I have had the flu or something for the past two days. The fever, chest aches, body aches, congestion...and so on. I still feel horrible tonight."

Jackie felt the worst she had in years! She asked if we should move the practice triathlon to two days before her actual race. I told Jackie the rule of thumb is she should not exercise with a fever.

I could not change my schedule. I had back-to-back clients and I was leaving for Florida. Kasey had arranged for someone to watch her children, was planning not to do her favorite yoga class, and the list went on. We were all set for the practice triathlon with Jackie and had now been thrown a big curve. But, the client comes first. We ask for 24 hours notice for cancellations or rescheduling to allow us to make other client appointments. I didn't know if Kasey would even get this email in time to change her schedule.

10

Doing Too Much

I did not recommend going through with the practice triathlon because it would be too close to the real race and Jackie was too sick. I couldn't believe she was even considering it. I told her to listen to her body. If her goal was to do the real triathlon, she should save her energy.

> *"I hope and pray that I won't miss the actual race,"* Jackie coughed, *"but I will if I don't get better. Just pray it doesn't happen. I've been waiting for this for four months!"* She was so disappointed.

Jackie had waited until the very last minute before she could admit that she might not make it. Jackie, like many women, was desperately trying to do everything she had planned on doing, even at the risk of jeopardizing her health. I'm guilty too. I remember having stitches in my knee (I had some scar tissue removed), and took a body sculpting class. I was on my side doing leg lifts, which was ridiculous! I was in my 30s then, now, in my 40s I know better.

It is tough when you train for something, look forward to it, and then get sick. Many times it crossed my mind that Jackie might have over trained. I didn't know for sure. I do know there was a lot of sickness going around so it may have just been bad timing.

Jackie had gone to the doctor and did have the flu. The only thing she could do is rest up for the race. Cheryl reassured me that if Jackie did decide to do the triathlon, she promised to take good care of her and give me a full report when I got back in town.

Honey, If You Can Do It...

It was Sunday, March 2nd — race day. No phone calls or email from Jackie, so the race was on!

Jackie's husband and kids drove her to the indoor triathlon. She said, "I was so nervous. I thought my husband was about ready to push me out of the car. He was trying to pump up my confidence, but I was having none of it." Jackie was just in a bad mood, nervous and afraid of failure. The thought running through her head was, "Todd and the kids are going to witness me fail!" Jackie didn't know what to expect and just wanted to get one triathlon under her belt.

Unfortunately, Cheryl got lost on the way to the event and by the time she got there the race had already begun. She was disappointed because the swimming was already done and Jackie had transitioned to the bike. Cheryl really was hoping to see the swimming. She was surprised that it was such a low-key event. The athletic club was so large, the competitors pretty much blended in with the members of the club who were working out. It was a beautiful facility; it just didn't feel like there was a race going on.

For Jackie the swimming had been a blur and the breathing had been hard for her. "I remember watching the first wave of people jumping in the pool," Jackie recalled. "I watched a girl doggy paddle the whole time. I was watching for people who could possibly do worse than me. Horrible, huh? Not that I wish bad things on other people, but I wanted to make sure I was okay. I wanted to verify in my mind that I didn't have to be a super athlete to do a triathlon. I just had to be the best that I wanted myself to be! I jumped in the pool and I did my best."

Jackie's husband, Todd, felt Jackie had struggled with the swimming. The club volunteer, who kept track of her distance for each heat, felt Jackie was slow and steady and she was quite impressed when she heard that Jackie had just learned how to swim correctly. Jackie swam 12 laps and then transitioned to the stationary bike. The club volunteer was wonderful, very attentive to Jackie, brought her water and apple juice, rubbed her back and cheered her on.

Cheryl found Jackie on a bike; she seemed focused and determined, her pace was good and steady. Jackie listened to music and she seemed to concentrate on the exercise and not the room around her.

> *"I got on the bike and just started spinning my*
> *legs as fast as I could," Jackie told me.*

"I set the resistance to one or two and thought the faster I spin, the faster I'll go. It just didn't seem to work that way. People were still going a further distance than I was." What Jackie didn't realize at the time was that using a higher resistance would have actually given her more distance. Lesson learned. Toward the end of the 30 minutes Jackie seemed to struggle with breathing and she told Cheryl her chest was tight from being sick. She rode for 6.10 miles.

During the transition between the bike and the treadmill, Jackie was coughing a little and told Cheryl her breathing was a bit off. She had a chance to talk to Cheryl before the next event and told her the swimming had scared her the most. She wasn't worried about the treadmill, though, because she knew she could walk if she needed. She drank some water and headed for the treadmill.

Jackie started out at a jog. For the most part she kept a steady pace although she did speed up a few times and slow to a walk at times to catch her breath. She listened to music and didn't talk during the run. Jackie hit her first mile at 11.2 minutes and finished around 1.73 miles in the allotted 20 minutes.

Later, Jackie said, "It wasn't too bad. I ran next to a guy who ran an 8-minute mile and next to a woman who was 20 years older than me. She ran a 10-minute mile, but I just did my best.

"When I was done, I couldn't believe that I even did it. I still had more training to do, but to do all three events after never doing anything at all felt awesome! I finally showed myself that I was making progress.

"I remember this woman grabbed my face and told me, 'Honey, if you can do it, I know anyone can.' I know it seems like a funny thing for her to say, but she said it because I was still getting over the flu. She felt if someone could be getting over the flu and still do a triathlon, then maybe more people could do this if they put their excuses aside."

When she finished running Jackie pretty much stopped cold — not much of a cool down. She didn't look well to Cheryl at first, but she was smiling and glad it was over. Jackie sat down on the end of the treadmill and said she would probably sleep for the rest of the day. Her family sat with her and gave her a hug. When Cheryl asked the kids if they were proud of their mom, they both smiled and nodded.

Cheryl asked Jackie if she would do it again. Jackie said she was really glad she did this race, even though she had been sick. Jackie wasn't afraid of doing it again — if she could do it after the flu, there was nothing to fear when she was healthy.

Cheryl told me she felt Jackie's health held her back a little, but it seemed she made the right choice to go through with the triathlon. It boosted her confidence. "I think she'll be great at the next one," Cheryl recounted. "While watching her I didn't see someone who had been sick — I saw a very focused and determined athlete. I was inspired just watching her, and even my daughter who was with me was so motivated she wanted to go home and set up exercise stations like the triathlon," Cheryl said.

I was sorry I missed Jackie's first triathlon, but she filled me in, "I was on the bike and Cheryl said, 'You know what Linda would say, listen to your body.' I laughed because just as she was saying it, the same thought was running through my head! I think she said it when I looked kind of shaky. It was like you were there with me!"

Next Step — The Bike

With her first triathlon under her belt, Jackie's confidence was soaring.

> *"What I learned from this whole triathlon experience was to just show up!" she told me. "I put it on my schedule. Just like when I told myself I was going to go to a cycling class. I wrote it down and showed up. Okay, okay, not always, especially that darn 5:30 am class, but more times than not."*

Due to the fact that she completed the indoor triathlon after being so sick, Jackie knew she could tackle bigger and better races.

Two days after the triathlon I saw Jackie at our March BPW meeting. Her hair was adorable; it was curly from a new perm. A professional organizer gave the presentation that evening and Jackie said, "I'm not the most organized person." Many people in the audience nodded their heads because they could relate to her comment.

Jackie was finishing up the meeting when she announced to the group that she had just completed her first triathlon. Everyone clapped. She told them about the journey she had taken so far. After completing the triathlon and receiving her medal, she felt all her hard work had been validated and she was in really good shape now.

Someone asked about her preparation, so Jackie described her training; she swam one or two times a week, biked three times, and ran one to two times each week. They all laughed when she reminded them that when she first started training, she couldn't swim, bike or run, but signed up for a triathlon anyway at my suggestion. Jackie added that she was just getting over the flu when she did the race, but because she had signed up for it she was determined to go through with it.

After the meeting, Jackie and I spoke and decided it was time for her to get outside and ride a bike to start training for her next triathlon. I offered for her to borrow a bike from me since she still didn't have one. She accepted. I told her to pick up a helmet since she would be required to have one of her own for her next race.

I coordinated with Kasey and found a date which would work for all of us in early April. I told Kasey that I had a mountain bike for Jackie to use. Since Jackie hadn't biked in years I preferred she mess up my inexpensive bike rather than Kasey's new racing bike she had invested in for triathlons. I also owned a hybrid mountain bike which I would use. The result was we had three different bikes for Jackie to try so she could feel the differences. When Jackie tried my mountain bikes, I suspected she would want to buy a racing bike like Kasey's.

I had purchased a bike carrier so I could transport the bikes to Jackie's house. Since I have a convertible, I usually have the top down and put my bike in the car. Considering the temperature was only 40 degrees, I didn't really want to do this.

As is often the case, things don't always work out as planned. I ended up taking the bike carrier off my car because it wasn't installed properly — it moved as soon as I touched it. All I needed to do was scratch my trunk with my bike carrier and spend hundreds in repairs. I had no choice. I had to put the top down in the car and squeeze the two mountain bikes in the back seat. Did I mention it was 40 degrees that morning with no sun? It was very cold! Thank goodness for my ear covers and gloves. I drove with the heat on full blast — I must have looked like a wild woman!

I arrived at Jackie's house and Kasey pulled in right behind me. We were dressed for the weather but Jackie wasn't. She wore a light shirt, a light zip-up sweatshirt, and capri pants. We suggested she change so she put on long pants.

"I have my helmet," Jackie said, "but I haven't been on a bike since high school." As she showed us a scar on her knee from a fall off a bike when she was a kid she said, "I'm not afraid to ride despite my not-so-great bike-riding history."

In training for the triathlon, she had been taking cycling classes at the YMCA; she would soon see just how different riding outside really is.

We headed outside. Brrr, cold, overcast and no sun at all. I explained that the progression for Jackie would be to ride my old mountain bike first, then my hybrid mountain bike and finally Kasey's racing bike (I didn't tell her how heavy the mountain bikes were). Before Jackie got on the old mountain bike, I told her the bike was sentimental to me because it was the one I used to help train a client — one who was once 300+ pounds. He now competes in full Ironman triathlons! (Those include a 2.4-mile swim, 115-mile bike, and a full marathon of 26.2 miles.) Jackie and I went over the gears, how to shift, and the brakes. I asked her which was the flattest way to go out of her driveway and she said to the left. Left it was — we were off.

Jackie started out okay though she was apprehensive, which was perfectly understandable. I rode next to her and talked gears, low numbers make her spin faster and help her get up hills. Higher gears will help her go faster on a straightaway. Kasey talked to Jackie about cadence, making sure she kept the same cadence going up hills, down hills and when riding straight. Understanding the gears would be critical when Jackie raced.

After one loop around the neighborhood, Jackie wanted to go in and get a coat. She couldn't find one so she opted for a scarf which she tied around her neck to keep it warm. This time, we all turned right out of her driveway which meant we had a steeper hill to climb. She could feel it on the old mountain bike and worked the gears as she climbed.

When we reached the top it was time for a bike swap. Jackie took over the hybrid mountain bike, which had a padded seat. The gears were different from the mountain bike; they changed by turning the handlebar pad. I kept reminding her which brake was the back one because I didn't want her to squeeze only the front brakes and flip over the handlebars.

Kasey said, "We're not taking a break," so we didn't and continued on for a second lap. Going up the hill was very challenging for Jackie because the hybrid mountain bike was heavier and gears one through six didn't work. This meant Jackie was peddling in seventh gear, which was quite a workout. Jackie was breathing hard and her heart rate was up by the time we all got back to her house. Kasey wasn't really having a hard workout because she was riding her expensive racing bike. Yes, money does make a difference when it comes to equipment, which Jackie would soon find out.

We stopped at Jackie's house for a water break. She went inside to get a drink while Kasey and I stayed outside since we both had water bottles with us. This is also something Jackie learned: carry water with you on your bike. She told us she signed up for a triathlon in June in York, Pennsylvania. The swimming would again be in a pool, which made her happy. Jackie was not keen about swimming in a pond so I suspect she chose this one intentionally because of the pool. The bike and run would be outside this time. We were getting closer to a more traditional triathlon.

We made the final bike switch, which meant Jackie would be riding Kasey's bike. Kasey explained how to use the toe clips, gears and brakes. Kasey's racing bike was totally different from the two mountain bikes so they spent some time with it before we started. The toe clips were new to Jackie. Kasey told her some people use special shoes for the bike portion of a triathlon. When Jackie asked if she could run in those special shoes Kasey explained the bike shoes were only for biking. No cutting corners there, the right equipment for the right job would be critical!

We rode off, but Jackie was having problems getting a foot in the toe clips. Kasey held on to the bike while Jackie was on it then slowly moved away. Jackie struggled some with the gears and brakes, even started in a crouched-down position then moved to a more upright position. We encouraged her not to get frustrated, reminding her that once she purchased her own bike, she would get used to it and all of its gadgets.

Going up the small hill was a breeze for Jackie this time, but Kasey and I struggled on the mountain bikes. Especially Kasey since she rode the hybrid bike which left her in seventh gear. We turned around and Jackie had to use a car door handle to steady herself while she got her foot in the toe clip. As we went up the big hill Jackie didn't have to do much work but I had to stand up to keep up with her. Kasey stayed in a seated position and I had Jackie look back to see how far Kasey was from us. I also asked Jackie to listen to how Kasey and I were breathing. I pointed out that if we had been wearing heart rate monitors, Kasey and my heart rates would have been a lot higher than Jackie's.

> "I can see how the wrong bike puts you at a disadvantage," Jackie said.

Feeling the major differences in the bikes was critical for Jackie. She now understood what was unique about all three. With this experience she could start to form opinions on what she wanted in a bike. I told her to make sure she tries one before buying it and to check the return policy. Jackie commented that Kasey's brakes hurt her thumbs. We want Jackie to be 100 percent comfortable with her new bike. She would have to take this into consideration while shopping. I reminded her that buying a bike to use in a triathlon will be an investment, unlike buying an inexpensive bike to ride around the neighborhood.

We stood and stretched in her driveway. "I feel it in my quads," Jackie said. She takes cycling classes so I reiterated why it's important for her to train outside, where she'll be competing. Otherwise her muscles won't be prepared.

We did six loops which was around three miles. Her next triathlon will include a 12-mile bike ride. Kasey suggested to Jackie she should train for 15 miles. She also told her to strive for a certain amount of time in addition to the distance. For example, it took Kasey 35 minutes to finish the bike portion of her triathlon so Kasey trained for 45 minutes.

June 29th was Jackie's triathlon in York and Kasey felt Jackie would be ready considering it was still three months away. Jackie was talking about the training involved and I encouraged her to keep scheduling it into her day, like she had been doing.

As we continued to chat outside, Jackie talked about the Schuylkill River.

> *"There's a triathlon on August 3rd I'm considering," she said, "I'm addicted to triathlons now. Are you shocked? Your pool-swimmer considering tackling a very big river — it would be the ultimate accomplishment for me!"*

We left Jackie tired, but well informed. What we didn't tell her was next time I planned to bike for two laps and then run two laps.

I put the bikes in my car with the top down and it was now 41 degrees. As I drove off I thought to myself, who knew our "I don't know how to swim, I don't own a bike and I hate to run" girl might consider a triathlon in the Schuylkill River? That's the beauty of working with people to get them started on their journey. When they get a taste of success, their confidence builds and they really take off. This is why I love what I do!

Just Keep Racing

I checked in with Jackie to see how she felt after our bike ride. "I feel great," she told me. "Not sore or anything." There was no mention of her shoulder while we were biking and I made sure to remind Jackie not to push into the handlebars. I told her to relax her upper body and kept an eye on her form. The biking could have aggravated it, but Jackie didn't mention any shoulder pain. Yeah! This was great because we had a lot of work to do before her triathlon in June.

In April Jackie started to shop for a bike. The bikes she looked at ranged between $750-$1200 which was a big price difference. When Jackie consulted with Kasey and me on what she should be looking for, we told her she should look for a lightweight, reliable road model. The amount Jackie should invest in a bike would depend on how serious Jackie was about the sport. If she was looking to use the bike for recreational use and a few races a year, Kasey suggested she stick with a less expensive model. On the other hand, if Jackie was truly committed to competing in triathlons, she may want to invest more money. It was a decision she had to make for herself.

> Jackie chose the model for $750. She told me,
> "I'm getting more and more addicted to my
> training! I used to hate these three sports, now I
> hate it if I miss a day.

"Eventually I would like to do more races but I'm guessing the $750 model is a great bike to get me started. It's very lightweight. I also bought bike shorts and a top I can swim in; almost like a trisuit, but in two pieces.

Her enthusiasm was so exciting to witness. She had her bike. There was no stopping her now. This meant I would need to buy a good bike so I could keep up with Jackie and Kasey the next time we rode together! Otherwise I would have to drive my car behind those two on their speedy bikes.

I arrived at the May BPW meeting early. Jackie and I were alone for awhile, so I had a chance to hear about a mock triathlon she had done that day. She was last out of the pool, she told me, four minutes behind the others, but was able to make it up on her bike. Jackie said she passed women going up a hill because they were on mountain bikes. She really had an appreciation for the differences in bike models. She said, "I LOVE my new bike and try to get on it as much as I can."

We were trying to coordinate a group ride together again, but I received an email from Jackie saying, "What do you think about swimming instead of biking? Or doing both the same day? I'm horrible at the swimming. I don't have the endurance at all. I can go about six straight laps and then I'm out of breath. What do you think?"

Kasey and I were open to doing both the same day, but since Jackie was concerned about improving her stroke, we decided that she and Kasey should swim together first to focus on the swimming. They decided to meet for an early-morning swim.

I saw Jackie a couple days before their swim at the BPW Business Card Exchange. As always, she looked great. She was down to 129 pounds and looked fit. Jackie told me again how much she loves her new bike and how she had just been on it for a 10-mile ride. At the card exchange she was telling everyone about her triathlon and the training I had been doing with her. She told the group she now enjoys training five days a week and takes the weekends off to be with her family. She was so open to sharing!

On May 16th Jackie and Kasey swam together. Kasey did some research on improving strokes and gave Jackie several pointers. Overall, they swam 30 laps but didn't focus on endurance. They spent the entire time trying to improve Jackie's stroke.

The best part was that there were several other swimmers in the pool to use as examples. Two of the swimmers were awesome and one had a stroke very similar to Jackie's. As a result, Kasey was able to point out to Jackie what looked right and what could be improved. By the end, they had made a lot of progress and Jackie was very pleased.

Some of Kasey's pointers included:

1. Top of head should always point in the direction you want to swim. This is extremely important in open bodies of water.
2. Nose should point straight down and rotate from left to right when taking a breath. Pointing the nose toward the top of the water will lift the head and lower the hips, causing the body to drag in the water. This will greatly reduce swim speed and use additional energy.
3. Head should not be completely submerged in water. The top of the head should be slightly above water line and glide smoothly through water.
4. When taking a stroke, reach as far forward as possible to lengthen bodyline and maximize stroke.
5. When doing freestyle, elbow should exit water first before reaching forward. Hand should enter water with thumb down. *This really resonated with Jackie.*
6. Hand should skim top of water — not be lifted high in the air — while reaching forward in between each stroke. *This was another pointer that helped Jackie a lot.*

By the end of the hour, incorporating Kasey's pointers, Jackie had made vast improvements. In doing so, she didn't hurt her shoulder, which was huge. Kasey was impressed with the progress!

At the June BPW meeting, Jackie announced her next triathlon to the group. "Hey, is anyone coming to my triathlon? It's June 29th in York." Then she added that it would include a 500-meter swim (20 pool lengths), 15-mile bike race and 5K run.

Jackie filled me in on her solo training. She sometimes rode with the Tuesday 9:00 am or Thursday 5:30 am YMCA bikers outside.

"I felt for the girls on mountain bikes," she said. Jackie knows what it's like to ride a mountain bike and it was obvious she liked her new racing bike.

Then Jackie continued, "My...is sore." She pointed to the mid section of her groin area and I explained how some bikers have a tendency to push down in the front or should I say lean forward. She had on biking pants, which are padded, but I told her she would have to build up a tolerance in that area. It was a 15-mile ride so it was aggressive on her part and explained the tenderness. I was happy she actually rode with other people.

I sent Jackie an email to let her know that on the 29th, my stepchildren would be visiting from Tennessee and I wouldn't be able to make her triathlon. I asked her to send me information just in case my schedule changed. Too bad, I would have liked to be there to cheer her on.

In mid-June, Jackie attended a business card exchange which was followed by my "The Importance of Cross Training" presentation. Jackie had been attending my kickboxing classes at the YMCA, as well as riding bikes with her neighbors to the local tennis courts to play tennis. She had really grasped the concept of cross training.

> *Jackie enjoyed the presentation and said, "I love things like this — I love learning more about fitness!" She was telling people about her upcoming triathlon and was proud to say all the things that she does.*

She said she was biking today with the 5:30 am group. It was exciting to see someone genuinely interested in health and fitness, not just on the surface but deep down inside. "I wish I could do this full time and get paid for it," Jackie added.

That was the last time I saw Jackie until after her June 29th triathlon, when she filled me in. "I felt I did great!" Jackie proclaimed. "I did better than I thought I would. The swim was in a pool. They opened 10 lanes and every 30 seconds the next person would take off to swim. I was one of the last swimmers to jump in. They had us go up a lane and back down the other side and then under the rope to finish 10 complete laps. I was actually passing a few people. That impressed me, but when I got out I could barely breathe! I was so out of breath. It took me 15 minutes and 30 seconds to complete the swim.

"The bike took me 1 hour and 4 minutes to ride 15 miles. There were lots of pretty big hills, and a few long, windy hills going down. My chain fell off once. I had a major charley horse towards the end, but overall the bike ride was nice. I enjoy the bike!

"I walked probably the first couple minutes of the 5K run and I did it in 35 minutes. It was hard to transition from the bike to the run after that charley horse hit me, but once I shook it out and stretched it some, I ran the rest of the way without ever having to go back to walking. I was happy — it was the first time I did that.

"All in all, I was pleased with my results. I'll definitely do more races. I was in a great mood the rest of the day!"

I congratulated her and then filled Kasey and Cheryl in on Jackie's race. They had both invested time in Jackie and appreciated sharing in her accomplishment. I hated to miss it, but would have another opportunity to see Jackie compete because she had scheduled another triathlon on September 14th in Downingtown. This one would include a quarter-mile swim, 12.5-mile bike and a 2-mile run. If possible I really wanted to go witness the event. Jackie would be doing her first full outdoor triathlon *and* she would be swimming in a lake.

She had officially caught the triathlon bug!

Jumping In A Lake

It was hard to believe it was already September and time for Jackie to compete in another triathlon. As it turned out, I was finally able to clear my calendar to attend. I asked Jackie if it would make her nervous to have me there. "It will probably make me do better knowing people may be watching," she told me and then added, "I think Todd and the kids are going too. Todd makes me nervous! I just want to do well in front of him."

A few days before the race, Jackie's bike had a little accident. It fell off the garage wall during the night and slipped under her car. In the morning, not knowing it was there, she backed over the front wheel. She took it in to get repaired and luckily was able to pick it up before race day. Of all things to happen — she drove over her bike!

I offered to drive Jackie to the race unless she wanted to go alone. I gave her the choice; some athletes like the time to focus on the race and prefer to travel alone, while others like some distraction. She decided to meet me there because Todd and the kids were going with her.

This triathlon was especially significant for Jackie, as she would be swimming in a lake. It shocked me that my pool-swimmer put her fears of snakes aside! She would be in the water at 7:40 am. I think she even surprised herself with her decision.

> *"I never thought anyone in this world could make me want to jump in a LAKE! And you succeeded!" Jackie exclaimed.*

Early that morning, I set out to meet Jackie at the triathlon. All night I had left the house air conditioner on because it had been so hot, and it was still running when I left in the morning. It was dark at 6:15 am, it was 73 degrees, very foggy, and the humidity was at 90 percent. Oh, was it muggy!

Earlier in the week someone asked me if I competed in triathlons and I said no because I swim like a stone. I sink to the bottom. I thought about this conversation as I was driving to Jackie's triathlon — why couldn't I do a triathlon? I train others to do them so why not me? I should set this as a goal before I turn 50. I could work on my swimming. Biking would not be an issue, but the big problem would be running. I have had several knee surgeries over the years and one was not totally successful, ending my running career. Maybe I could run again; I'd have to try. I toyed with the idea. Jackie was inspirational!

As I continued my drive, I turned on the radio to get the weather report. "Hazy, hot and humid," it stated, "with the temperature reaching a possible record-breaking 92 degrees." Thank goodness Jackie was starting out early because it was shaping up to be a nasty day for a race. I drove on knowing Jackie was already there setting up her gear.

I approached Marsh Creek State Park just after 7:00 am where people were running up the street to warm up their muscles. They did not have to run far to warm up because it was so humid outside. Seeing all the different shapes and sizes and ages of the competitors excited me. Almost anyone can do a triathlon; there are distances for everyone.

It was 30 minutes before Jackie would swim and I had to find her in a crowd of 600 competitors and countless spectators. Not an easy task! I waited by the transition area because she'd have to pick up her goggles and mandatory swim cap there. Still no Jackie. Where was she? Maybe the bathroom. The line was long even though they had lots of port-o-potties. Many competitors go one last time before heading down to the swim area.

Finally I spotted her. She looked so frazzled, almost running toward the transition area, which was now practically empty because the competitors were already on their way to the lake. She was saying something to Todd when I saw her.

I hugged her hello, she gave each of the kids a kiss goodbye and we walked down to the lake together. She was a nonstop chatterer. "It's crowded!" she noted. She was right, there were close to 600 athletes participating. I asked what she had for dinner last night and she said broccoli and something else. She wasn't sure what to eat before a race. I would really need to talk with her about what to eat before a race. Evidently something had happened at her last race as a result of her dinner the night before, which left her uncertain. If we had been working together on a regular basis, I could have filled her in on these important matters. Bodies need fuel to perform well in competition! The good news was she did have a protein shake and a banana that morning.

It was an amazing feeling to walk with Jackie to the lake. I was taking pictures of her all along the way and even took a picture of a sign the state park had posted stating, "No Swimming In The Lake." Only during closely supervised triathlons was swimming allowed.

The family caught up with us and she kissed them one more time. She commented on her tinted goggles, "I shouldn't have bought these," she said. On an overcast day, she wouldn't need tinted goggles, but I felt she would be okay.

Then Jackie added, "I haven't ridden my bike in a while." It was not a good time to mention this and it concerned me, but she had a good reason — running over her bike — so she couldn't ride it for a few days.

Referring to the big group that was already in the water, Jackie said, "I don't want to be in the middle of the pack. Is that okay?" She wanted to be at the end or near a side, just not in the middle of the pack of swimmers. I assured her it was fine. I kept reminding her she was there to have fun and to learn what to do for her next triathlon.

> *I watched her put on her swim cap and walk into the water. "I've gotten better at swimming," she said as she walked into the lake.*

Jackie was a woman who did not like to swim anywhere but a pool and there she was, wading into some very deep water. The kicker? She had just learned she would have to tread water out there until they called her age group to start. If you think about it, it is a truly awesome feat! She didn't like snakes and she didn't like murky water, but there she was, treading water in a lake. It gave me chills.

I called out to Jackie to ask about the temperature of the water. "It's cool!" she said. Some people had on wet suits but Jackie didn't need one. She got over the temperature quickly because of her nerves.

I was on the deck with the starter when he said, "Three minutes." There was Jackie's yellow bathing cap bobbing in the lake. It was exciting! "Two minutes!" "One minute!" I was jumping up and down. She was almost ready to swim. "Ten, nine, eight, seven, six, five, four, three, two, one, go." Wow!

Jackie was wearing a bright pink top so it was easy to spot her in the water. The tinted goggles helped too. As the yellow bathing caps slowly moved forward, I saw Jackie on her back. Was she floating? Then, I saw her doing a side crawl. Swimming wasn't her strong point and that's okay because everyone has one weakness in this type of race. She was on her back again, very unusual for a triathlon. I was able to follow her along the quarter-mile swim because they were relatively close to shore. I kept yelling, "Go Jackie! Come on Jackie!" in the hope she could hear me. What I really wanted her to hear was that she was heading to shore and she shouldn't be. Being on her back, she wasn't able to see she was off course. Finally, she looked up and corrected her course.

> She later admitted, "I was afraid the official with the whistle was going to disqualify me for swimming too close to the buoys! I did panic a little — was unsure what to do because I was so nervous, but I just calmed myself down. That's why I went to my back, because I needed time to breathe, take a deep breath, and release some nerves."

Orange bathing caps, the group behind her, were swimming by her. It was okay because it was after all, her first lake swim. And, she was using both her left and right sides to breathe, which was new to her.

Jackie slowly emerged from the water and you could tell it was tough. The quarter-mile swim got to her and she looked tired. According to my watch, her swim took around 14 minutes.

When she walked up the ramp toward the transition area, I yelled, "You did it!" and high-fived her. Actually it was a low-five because she was tired and her hand didn't go up that high. Her only words to me were, "It was hard!" That was obvious.

Prior to getting in the water Jackie said she was going to take it easy on the swim because she heard the bike trail was hilly. Her plan was to pace herself and I reassured her she'd do okay on the swim and the bike. However I don't think she realized how tiring the swimming would be.

I ran up the hill so I could get a picture of her coming out of Transition One (T1), but didn't see Jackie. T1 was where the competitors could get out of their wet gear if they wanted to and change into something dry. There they put on shoes, socks, a helmet, ate, drank, put on their number and whatever else they chose to do. Some people wet their feet then dry them again so they wouldn't have to ride their bikes with sand in their shoes.

I was afraid I had missed her, but she was still in T1 eating something, drinking something, putting on her paper number and getting herself together. Eventually she appeared. "Come on Jackie!" I yelled to try and move her along. It may have taken three minutes to transition; I would have to check her stats after the race.

When she finally did walk up the hill with her bike, the others were running their bikes up the hill. I said, "You just swam in a lake!" That brought a smile to her tired face.

She mounted her bike and began the 12-mile, very hilly bike ride. Fortunately, although it was humid, it was overcast. "I haven't ridden in a while." Jackie's words echoed in my mind because her lack of training could catch up with her. The bike ride would take about 50 minutes so I sat down and wrote notes on everything that had happened so far.

As I wrote, I could see the first racer arrive at the dismount area. A worker stood there shouting to him, "Get ready to dismount! Get ready to dismount!" The man got off his bike, ran it into Transition Two (T2), hooked his bike on the rack, changed shoes, threw off his helmet, then began running two miles.

To help pass the time, Jackie's daughter was also on a bike. She looked cute wearing her little pink helmet on her little pink bike. Todd told me he was getting a workout just chasing her around.

The first woman came into T2 at 8:25 am and there was quite a cheer for her. The color of the bathing cap dictated the age and gender of the swimmers they sent out in waves. It was easy to tell who was who when they were in the water, but once they were out and had on helmets, you couldn't tell at all. Was this woman in Jackie's wave or did she go out at 7:30 am? I didn't know.

It was fun to sit there and watch the bodies. Some were so muscular and toned while others were soft and fluffy. The bikes were fascinating. They ranged from the dreaded heavy mountain bike to the super sleek bike with the clips attached to the pedals. Even the helmets were different; some very aerodynamic while others were of the less-expensive variety.

As we waited, Todd mentioned that Jackie talked about doing a relay triathlon where someone would swim, she would bike and then someone else would run. Heck, I'd volunteer for the bike part, but it sounded like cycling was Jackie's favorite too.

It was getting close to the time when Jackie would be coming into T2. Todd, the kids and I were looking for her. "Is that Mom? Is that Mom?" the kids kept asking. Fortunately, Jackie's pink shirt made it easy to spot her and we did see her come in. "It takes courage to enter in a triathlon," Todd said. He had that right!

The bike took Jackie around 50 minutes as she had predicted it would. She looked so tired. Jackie dismounted and then slowly walked her bike down the hill into the T2 area. Other athletes were running their bikes down, but I'm glad Jackie didn't. Competing in anything, especially triathlons, you have to learn about your body, your equipment, the race, everything. You could tell which of the competitors were seasoned, they knew exactly what to do. For example, the vets rode their bikes until they absolutely had to get off to dismount, while the newer racers dismounted early and lost time. In a triathlon, time counts from the moment you take your first stroke in the water. Transition times need to be kept as brief as possible.

Jackie missed her assigned row to hang her bike up so she had to backtrack. Each athlete was given a number to wear which corresponded to where they were to hang their bike and put their clothes in the transition area. She ate something, drank something, took off her helmet, hung up her bike, and headed out. The T2 was about a minute and a half; it was much faster than T1, which was typical.

I took pictures of Jackie coming in from her bike, while she was in T2 and then heading out for her run. There was no smile on her face when I yelled, "Good job!" She just looked at me. Unfortunately, the sun came out. It was already humid but with the sun, it was terrible. They were running right into it. Luckily, for this particular race, the running portion was only two miles — I don't think she would have wanted to run three — but, it was an uphill run on tired legs.

Jackie's run lasted twenty minutes in full sun. I was yelling as she approached the line of flags leading up to the finish line. I high-fived her as she ran by. She was one tired puppy, but that puppy had just completed her first outdoor triathlon!

I ran along side of her and tried to get a picture of her crossing the finish line, at about an hour and forty minutes, maybe an hour and forty-two. I immediately found her, hugged her and she sat down.

> *"I know I shouldn't, but I have to sit down," she*
> *mumbled. She was shaking; her hands and even*
> *her forehead were trembling.*

I told her she had taken her body to where it had never gone before, but even through the fatigue, I could tell she was happy. She was shaking but happy. The family found us and kissed her. Because she was so shaky, Jackie couldn't hold her water. She even asked me to open the power drink because she didn't have the strength to do it. I was glad to oblige.

> *"I'm proudest of this one because I had to push myself," Jackie said.*

Even though this was her third triathlon, the others were inside, the swim was in a pool and they weren't as crowded. This was a real race. Eventually my goal would be for her do a Sprint Triathlon: approximately a quarter-mile swim, 15-mile bike and 5K (3.1 miles) run, but I didn't tell her this then.

Jackie continued, "I did better on the swim than the last race, by a minute and a half." It was obvious she was proud of beating her own time from the last race. "For the run," she added, "I walked up a few hills, and asked some guy if he'd carry me." The important thing was that she completed the race. "Thank you for coming!" she said. We hugged and I told her again how proud I was of her.

Then an announcement came over the loud speaker to clean out the transition area for the award ceremony. "Did you win?" her daughter asked. "Did you win an award?" I responded to her that her mom was definitely a winner because she finished the race. I hoped the pictures would turn out of her in the transition area with the kids. It was adorable to watch. As she was cleaning out her space, four women were just finishing their bike ride.

Jackie said she didn't want to eat because she was afraid of getting sick. She was now standing, but still shaking. From the food offered she opted for a mini muffin, but couldn't hold on to it. I have to say it was unusual for someone to shake that much, but Jackie had really pushed her body. She said once she sits down in the car and calms down, she would be all right and I believed her.

> *Despite her exhaustion, Jackie stated, "I'm going to do all three triathlons again next year! And, I might do another one too! I'm hooked! I like to see my kids' faces when I cross the finish line! It keeps me going knowing I'll see them when I'm done — what a great motivator."*

Jackie then asked me to tell Todd about my client who was over 300 pounds when I started to work with him. Since losing one hundred pounds, he now competes in full Ironman triathlons. Those include a 2.4-mile swim, 115-mile bike, and a full marathon — 26.2 miles, I explained. "You won't see me doing that. No way!" Jackie commented.

As we walked to our cars together, she still couldn't hold her water bottle or gym bag because she was still shaky. I wanted her to get in the car and sit down. Todd took her bike up the long hill to the car. We parted at 9:50 am and I was so glad I was able to witness her race. How exciting! I couldn't wait to see the pictures.

Her son had a football game that afternoon. Because she was so exhausted I wondered if Jackie would go. I hoped she would do additional stretches to relax her much-used muscles. She would need to hydrate as well.

When I got home, it was hot and I was grateful Jackie didn't have to compete in the nasty, humid weather. I took a walk, even jogged a bit to see how my knees would feel. Sadly, they hurt so I stopped. I tried again fifteen minutes later, but had to stop because of sharp pains in one knee. It was official; my desire to do a triathlon would not be fulfilled. It would have been great to do one. Being the optimistic person I am, I knew I could still compete in a relay so I would have to look into that. Until then, I would live vicariously through Jackie and my other triathlon clients. It had been such a good day!

The times were posted on the triathlon website later that day so I checked Jackie's stats. The swim took Jackie 14:04, time in T1 was 2:24, the 12.5-mile bike took 52:10, time in T2 was 1:12 and the two-mile run took 22:30. The grand total time was 1:32:18. In her age and gender group, 35-39, she finished 38th out of 55, and overall she placed 387th out of 497 racers completing the triathlon.

The winner was a 20-24 year old male, finishing the race in 55:02. The first female to cross the finish line, a 25-29 year old, finished in 1:03:29 — the 29th person to finish. The last person to finish the race was a woman, age 30-34, in a time of 2:28:16. I bet she was on top of the world! She too had completed a triathlon.

Jackie felt really good after the race and told me what a great day it was for her too. She had her triathlon, Nathan had an awesome football game and they met a friend for dinner. "My butt and legs were tight, but I felt great." She was pleased with her results, but could easily see where she could improve. She planned to spend some time working on those areas and start competing again the following year.

"When I look back from where I started knowing nothing at all, to where I am now, I am at the point where I can pat myself on the back for it," Jackie emotionally explained to me. She went on to say, "Some people move their way up to their best really fast and some at a slower pace. And when I say the best, I mean the best that I want to be. It doesn't mean it is better than someone else. It just means better than where I was before. I am at MY best at this moment, and in six months, I'll even be better. It's exciting!

> "Instead of just dropping fat off my body, I'm leaving behind a different me. I feel I am a stronger and more confident person. Triathlons have become a part of who I am. I could never give that part of me up now. I love that part of me!

> "Now, I am beginning to see why you recommended triathlons to me. I told you I wanted something to accomplish. I was exercising and never feeling like I was getting anywhere or feeling any sense of accomplishment. You knew exactly what I needed before I even knew it. Not in a million years would I have ever wanted to swim, bike and RUN!

> "I know too many people who give up on themselves too early. They sit around worrying whether or not they should do something or if they shouldn't. I always hear excuses on why they cannot do this or that, or who tells them that they can't. Well maybe they can't today, but I would tell them to never say 'never.' When

I was younger, the only time you would have caught me running anywhere was running away from my friend's younger brother chasing me with a worm! You should have seen how fast I could go then!

"I fought with myself a lot this past year while training. I asked myself why I was doing this? Today, I figured it out."

Jackie Gets A Book Offer

For the next couple of months after her emotional triathlon, I only saw Jackie sporadically at various networking events. Her smile was always infectious and she spoke enthusiastically to everyone who would listen about her addiction to triathlons. She told them about her plans to repeat all three triathlons from the previous year and maybe add a fourth, an all-female triathlon. As she spoke to them, I could see in their faces that she was inspiring them to perhaps work out as well.

The holidays came and went and it was December 29th before we had a chance to sit down and talk. I asked Jackie to meet me at a local coffee shop and she agreed, with no questions asked.

As we stood waiting to get our coffee, I asked Jackie if she wondered why I wanted to see her. "To stop doing triathlons?" she questioned. She was actually afraid I was going to tell her triathlons were bad for her. Her next guess was that I was going to ask her to help someone else train for a triathlon.

She was shocked when I told her the real reason — I wanted her to be the subject of my next book.

> *"That would be awesome!" she blurted and continued, "A book about someone who had gone from nothing to this? Maybe I could help motivate others." She was really excited and added with a smile, "I'm an open book!"*

I asked her to write down her thoughts, starting now and going back to when we first met. We would then chronicle her second year of races. It was obvious she was excited.

"The goal now is to beat my times from last year's triathlons." Jackie said. "Last year, the goal was to FINISH the triathlon. I can't believe I accomplished that! NOW, the new goal is finish with a better time."

As we were pulling out of the driveway of the coffee shop, Jackie was already on the phone with her mother about her news. Her mom laughed and shared in her excitement as she headed home to tell Todd. Jackie hoped he'd have the same reaction.

Todd's response was a little less optimistic and she questioned why she let him in on the day's events. He joked with her how she better hurry up and get in shape. With this she went from being excited to a little worried.

"Hmmm, what if I look like a fool?" Jackie asked herself. "Should I get to the gym more? Should I skip the eggnog on New Year's? Or should I just go for it one last time before the New Year and drink all the eggnog I want! My husband is very realistic — he's good for getting me to think about what could go wrong.

> *"But for some reason I still tend to move forward," she said. "If we all held ourselves back because of what others thought of us, then we would never go anywhere."*

Jackie's inner dialogue convinced her that agreeing to be the subject of a book was definitely a good thing.

In January the reality of the book offer really sunk in when Jackie had the opportunity to meet Suzanne, the subject of my first book, *Journey to Fitness — Chronicles of a Working Woman*. It was at a business card exchange when "Book Two" was introduced to "Book One." The look in Jackie's eyes was priceless; she was in awe of Suzanne.

As people started to trickle into the business card exchange, Jackie and Suzanne were sharing stories of how I got them to do things they never would have done or thought they could do. I see the potential in people. In Suzanne's case, a 20-minute workout erased 30 years of self-doubt. Power. In Jackie's case she liked to work out, but only did so sporadically. So having Jackie schedule exercise into her day and giving her a big challenge like a triathlon, seemed the right thing to do. I knew they both had it in them; the challenge was getting them to believe in themselves.

It was great to step back and listen to the two women tell others what they had accomplished. "When Linda looks at you, you just do it," Jackie said. What shocked me was when she added, "I stop running when I see Todd or someone else going by because I don't feel I'm a good jogger." Darn, we would still need to work on her self-confidence. On a brighter note, Jackie announced Todd had gotten her bike clips for Christmas and now she can go 150 rpm instead of 120 rpm. She's definitely getting faster and more comfortable on her bike.

Suzanne and I were signing my book that evening, so Jackie had the opportunity to see Suzanne in the spotlight. I told Jackie that this time next year, people would want her autograph. "Will I have the paparazzi after me too?" she joked. "Yes," I said, "but they won't be in cars, they'll be on bicycles."

It was a magical evening for Jackie!

She's Got The Fever

Jackie continued to train for her second year of triathlons. Her goal was to bike two times per week, swim two times per week, and then run three times per week. It seemed like a lot, but if she paired activities up in the same day, she could swim and then go for a run, and complete both in one day. The YMCA triathlon class could get three activities out of the way another day, which basically left only one day to find time to run.

I told Jackie to plan her exercise, so every Sunday she sat down with her calendar and planned her workouts for the week. She was a very busy person so this was critical. She had her own cooking/kitchen tool business, sold real estate, volunteered at Nathan and Kayla's school, was President of the BPW group, and was a mom and took care of the house. She felt if she let anything slide she would make less money and her house would go to shambles. I'm not sure that would be true. I believed Jackie was a lot more organized than she gave herself credit for.

> *"The only thing that keeps me focused is exercise," Jackie explained to me.*

"It is the only thing in my life that I can go to and stay with until it is done. Believe me, things get done, but they all get done at the same time. If someone were watching me or if I were watching myself, it would be like watching four different movies at the same time. I'm sure most women feel the same way I feel. Exercise is my time though. If someone like me can find a way to fit it in and make the time to do it, then I know anyone can."

What A Difference

On February 8th, Jackie found herself on her way to repeat the indoor triathlon that started it all the year before. The difference? No flu and a lot more confidence!

The result? Jackie had really improved! Instead of 12 laps swimming, Jackie completed 16. She increased the bike portion of the race from 6.10 miles to a whopping 13.89 miles. "When the timers were coming around to get stats off of our bike, the woman's eyes got bigger when she saw how I did," Jackie proudly explained. "So, I started guessing that I did pretty well. Then everyone started commenting on it. I was so in the zone." She even increased her run from 1.73 miles to 1.88. Overall, she placed 15th out of 39 women and was happy to be in the top half of the racing results.

Jackie was really pumped up driving home from her race. While on the phone with her dad, telling him all about the race, she was pulled over by the police for driving too fast. She even told the officer all about her race. Jackie realized her races were athletic and she wasn't a race car driver. She would need to save her speed for her triathlons.

Later, Jackie reflected on what the last year had meant to her. "It clicked recently when I was thinking back," she told me.

> *"We blame others for making us feel a certain way, when nine times out of ten, it's our own inner demons talking to us instead."*

She was in some respects referring to Todd. In the beginning of her training she felt he had been overly critical, which is why she didn't want him to know about her training.

Todd would always tell Jackie she should do more than what she had just completed— four miles instead of three, for example. This frustrated Jackie and made her feel she wasn't good enough.

> *"But, you know what?" Jackie explained. "Do you remember when you came to the race at Marsh Creek State Park? Todd, Nathan, and Kayla drove me and were there to support me through the whole 'hottest day' ever event! That's when it hit me. I heard his voice while I was in the lake, I saw him smiling when I came down the hill with my bike, and then I got my hugs when I crossed the finish line after my run.*

> *"That race built my confidence in me. I was the one who thought I couldn't do it and I was the one who was embarrassed to run. All that time, I had it in my head how he was going to be embarrassed and that he didn't think I could do it. But I have found that I love him even more now because when I went to the last triathlon, he told me he was proud of me. Before I went out the door, he said 'Jackie, didn't you say you can do 15 laps in 10 minutes? Well, today do 16.' And guess what, I did it. I could not believe it. He pushed me because he knew I could do it.*

"We also kind of work out together now," Jackie continued. "We have workout DVDs and sometimes when we are on the same DVD, exercise together. He never would have worked out with me before because we both like to do it alone. I did the training and I did the triathlons but in a way, I think it made him happy too. Thank goodness for Todd. He is the other voice inside my head pushing me to do my best."

That realization was a huge turning point for Jackie in terms of self-awareness! She was finally starting to understand her own mindset in regards to her abilities and her feelings about triathlons.

Knowing What She Wants

In March, Jackie's cousin asked her to run a race with him in May. She was under the impression that it was a 10K (6.2 miles), which was a much longer race than she had been doing with the triathlons. Still, Jackie thought it would help her train and build her stamina. She signed up. Imagine her surprise when she found out it was a 10-mile race not a 10K!

> *"Could you imagine getting to the race to find out it was 10 miles and NOT 6.2 miles," Jackie laughed when she told me.*

"Running is really all in my head. I know I can run farther than I do, but I have it in my head I need to take breaks. My dad says if I keep going, I'll break past that. Just like the 'wall' runners talk about. I wonder how far I can run without stopping if I stop thinking about when my next break is!"

Jackie was actually considering running the race and asked for my suggestions on how to mentally prepare for it. "What do people think about when they run 10 miles? Is it relaxing for them?" she asked.

I told her she was a very brave woman to want to go from running 3.1 miles to running 10 miles and I believed she could do it. To eliminate injury though, I reminded her to go slow.

To begin training, I suggested Jackie pick an amount of time she wanted to run, 30 minutes for example, and then run it. Or she should pick a certain amount of miles, say four, and then run them. She could continue to do this until she's able to get both her body and her mind to run 10 miles. Her triathlons are that long overall and since she finishes them, she should be able to complete the total distance of a 10-mile run.

To help Jackie find ways to prepare mentally, I used my MRI experience as an example. People often say how horrible these procedures are and seek out coping methods. Many years ago I was in a serious car accident and was faced with several MRIs because of my head injuries. I found one way to get through the ordeal was through visualization. During a test I would go through the entire 45-minute long step routine I was teaching at the time. By the time I was through, the MRI would be over. I explained to Jackie how she could use a similar technique to prepare herself mentally. She could think of things that would keep her mind occupied while running. The entire time, however, she would still need to be listening to her body.

Running 10 miles would definitely be a mind game for Jackie. I suggested she start counting at zero, run to the first mile, then run to the second mile, then run to the third mile, etc., counting up as she clicks off the miles. At five miles, she would be halfway done and she could start counting backwards — only four more miles to go, only three more miles to go, then she would run for the finish line. She could also look for each water station as a treat or something worth running towards.

Jackie took my suggestions under consideration and started to train for the 10-mile race. Sadly, she began to experience knee pain and had to make a decision.

> *"My passion is to do the triathlons," she explained. "I decided that I did not want to risk injuring my knee for a 10-mile race I was not too happy about doing anyway. I realized how much I've grown to love doing the triathlons and that I am doing them to keep myself happy. All the self-talk and wondering if I am able to do such things are finally gone from my head. I KNOW I can do a triathlon now and my confidence is up. I am not ready to try a 10-mile race and risk taking away something I love to do, for something I was probably going to hate."*

Her newfound confidence was uplifting! Jackie had gone from not wanting to do a triathlon, to liking some parts of it, to now loving the entire race. Talk about coming full circle, what an amazing feeling it must be for her. It was just last year that Jackie didn't want to tell others or even her husband about possibly doing a race. Last year she was afraid for people to see her swim, she was nervous about biking, and she didn't want people to see her run. Wow! I was anxious to see what she would choose for her races this next year.

For the next two months, I only saw Jackie at networking events for a quick chat. It was not until May when we finally had a chance to get caught up. The evening was nice because it was the BPW Business Card Exchange, which meant we would have time to talk. As always, Jackie looked cute. She had on a form-fitting pair of pants and shirt, as only she could wear. She said she hadn't sent me any updates because there had been nothing to send. She was busy getting ready for her next triathlon in York, Pennsylvania on June 28th.

At one point Jackie said a YMCA lifeguard had noticed her stroke one day while she swam, and commented that she was taking her arm out of the water too soon. This prevented her from finishing the stroke and she wasn't getting the power she needed. "I remember Kasey telling me it should take me 19, 20 or 21 strokes to get across the pool," Jackie said. With the help of Kasey and the lifeguard's comments, instead of her 25 or 26 strokes she was able to get across the pool in 21, a major improvement and she could feel the difference. Jackie seemed happy and not nervous at all about her upcoming triathlon, which would have an indoor swim.

When I asked if she was doing Pilates and weight lifting, Jackie said she didn't have time because of all the triathlon training. I explained how important both were, in fact they could actually help improve her triathlon performance. Pilates would work her core and give her more power. Weight training would increase her overall strength and muscle tone and help her in all areas of a race.

We also talked about calories consumed, foods, and fiber. She didn't count calories but ate in moderation. She didn't totally eliminate any foods but again, she ate them in moderation. She tried to get enough fiber but not over do it. Fiber does have a tendency to bloat people so she knew to drink lots of water when consuming it.

Jackie seemed very comfortable. Relaxed. She was able to stand there and have people look at her while leading a conversation. She seemed confident. After our conversation that evening, Jackie decided to take my advice and try a Pilates class.

In June we met at a local coffee shop.

> *"The first year I had a fear of what to expect,"*
> *Jackie stated. "This second year, I have a fear*
> *of not beating last year's time."*

We talked about all the shapes and sizes of people who compete in triathlons and how they're deceiving because some are very strong though they may not look it. Those different shapes, sizes and ages beat her, even some people on mountain bikes. She said going forward she would pick someone ahead of her in her next race, and challenge herself to pass him or her. Great strategy!

Jackie also noted that many of the winners of her triathlons were in their 40s. I explained to her many women triathletes peak in their 40s. Jackie was still in her 30s and had only been competing for a year. I encouraged her to keep doing them. By age 40 she will have built such a solid foundation and would do really well in races too.

"I'd like to be thinner and have those six pack abs," Jackie added. Certainly she could have all of that, but it would mean a drastic cut in the food and drinks she's currently consuming. I asked her if she was willing to do these things and she responded firmly, "No!" As long as she was okay with how she looked and how she performed in races, she really didn't have to make any dietary changes.

> *We continued to talk about her next race. "The*
> *swimming worry is out of my mind," she said.*

This took me by surprise! I was glad I was sitting when she said it. But then she added, "I haven't been riding my bike as much this month. It's been raining a lot. I rode it the other day and my legs were tired." She agreed she needed to get back on her bike and ride, but at least she was seeing a big difference now that she was using biking shoes. Having the right equipment is so important!

Our hour was up as were our vanilla lattés. She was off to swim, and she had her bike in the car in case she had a chance to ride. I was off to meet another client. What a difference a year made. It was awesome to hear her talk about competing with such excitement in her voice. She truly had become a triathlete!

Something struck me as I was driving away; Jackie works three part-time jobs, has a husband and two young children participating in various activities, yet she still has time to train. My "disorganized" client had become very organized with her time. I didn't ask, but I bet she had scheduled exercise into her day this morning.

Lessons Learned

Jackie's triathlon in York, Pennsylvania was the morning of June 28th. She was awesome! The second time around she had more confidence and asked her family to be there with her. When she competed in this race last year she had a friend take her, figuring if she did poorly her friend would lie for her. Now, her children would have told her the truth. One year later, she knew she would be proud of the truth.

Jackie arrived early for her race. As a result she had plenty of time to set up — unlike the first year when she got lost and made it to the race just in time. Todd helped her take her bags and bike over to the transition area. Jackie placed her shoes on top of her towel, so she could quickly dry her feet after the swim before putting them on. She left her shoes untied so she could easily slip them on. When she questioned the woman next to her why she left her shoes tied, the woman told Jackie she just slipped them on that way.

Everyone has their own routine at a triathlon and there is always an opportunity to pick up tips from seasoned competitors to see what might work for you. Jackie placed a water bottle on her bike, two more by her shoes, and headed over to the pool for the indoor swim.

> *"I love the pool swim at this triathlon," Jackie stated. "There are races for everyone; pool, lake, ocean, river, but the pool is definitely my first choice. This year I felt so much more confident in the water. I passed people in their lanes, but no one passed me!"*

The previous year, it took Jackie 15 minutes and 30 seconds to complete the swim. She set her watch for 15 minutes to help judge her time this year. When she was out of the pool and already on her bike before the 15 minutes were up, she knew she was off to a great start.

Jackie started out a little slow on the bike. It was a very hilly course. She felt like it took forever to climb the hills, which seemed to her to be more like mountains. It took a lot of self-talk to get her to the top, but she didn't stop and was soon rewarded with a fast ride down the other side. Jackie loved to ride fast. "Some people are afraid to ride fast down the hills, but not me," she said. "I don't use my brakes at all except around turns and just love the chance to catch my breath before the next hill. The hills are tough, but I'd take a hilly course over a flat one any day." Despite a bit of a struggle with those hills, Jackie still managed to shave off some time. This helped her overall rank since she didn't decrease her running time as much as she wanted.

"When I got to the run, I was fading!" Jackie sighed. It was so hot and she felt like her legs were going to give out. At each water station she walked for a few minutes and just had to keep reminding herself she was almost done.

> *"You just know once you get to the run," she said, "you're at the end of your triathlon and the feeling of accomplishment will far outweigh the feeling you have right then...that your legs are about to fall off!"*

She had finished in around 35 minutes the first time she competed in the race, but only improved by a minute or so this time out.

When she crossed the finish line she almost burst out in tears. "I have no idea what the tears were for," she told me. "Glad it was done? Was I exhausted? Or maybe was I just happy to have beaten my time? Who knows?"

For those who have never trained for a triathlon or attended one, it can be tough to imagine how exhilarating it is. Jackie's tears resulted from everything she described. Emotions run very high at triathlons! Even though I don't compete in them, I get every bit as excited as the competitors and sometimes even more so, when I watch them.

Jackie was able to erase six minutes overall from the previous year's time. She could see the difference those six minutes would have made last year, moving her up 20 places. The fact that every second counts in a triathlon had finally sunk in.

The hard part about not working closely with her to train was we were unable to share with her all of these little tidbits along the way. I have noticed over the years, however, that when a competitor experiences this, he or she finally realizes how important every second or minute is in a race. Once they get it, they can start to find ways to take time off of their results.

Many years ago I watched one client compete in his first triathlon. He had just completed his swim and was getting ready for his bike in T1. I watched him slowly take off his wet suit, slowly peel a banana, slowly eat it, slowly put on his socks, and then slowly put on his sneakers. I kept yelling for him to hurry up and eat that darn banana on his bike. Another younger client thought T1 was a time to chat with her newfound friends. She was so busy talking to her new buddy that it seemed like she forgot about the race.

Recently, I started working with a couple who wanted to put up better times at their triathlons, in each part of the race. They told me that they spent six minutes in T1 at their last race. They were so happy to be done with the swim; they took their time savoring the moment. Needless-to-say, I practice transitions whenever possible with my clients.

Yes I Can

In July, Jackie and I met at a coffee shop so I could check on the training progress she was making for the Marsh Creek Triathlon. Jackie told me she wasn't really hungry or thirsty as we stood in line.

> *"These pastries don't appeal to me because I don't eat them anymore," Jackie said pointing to the treats in the case. "I'm also not a coffee drinker," she added. It was interesting to hear how her tastes had changed.*

While we were waiting for my iced coffee, I handed her the pictures of the Marsh Creek Triathlon from a year earlier. She studied them and really liked the one of her family. As she looked at them Jackie said, "I thought I'd take a week off from training after the last triathlon, but I've been traveling and on vacation so now it's been three weeks.

> *"We rode our bikes in Montana," she went on. "I thought I was in shape, but the altitude got to me. I had to push my bike up a hill."*

Jackie continued to look at the pictures of last year's triathlon. "All the professional photos they take of you at the triathlons aren't good. These are good."

Todd had told her that when other folks crossed the finish line, they hugged their families. Not Jackie. She laughed and mimicked herself saying, "Don't touch me. Get away from me. Mommy's hot so don't touch me right now." She hadn't realized it until Todd pointed it out and now she thought it was funny. I told her I'd be looking for it at her next race.

The swimming was no longer an issue for Jackie. She told me she was now breathing fine when she got out of the water. I was in shock! This from the woman who didn't know how to swim when I met her?

Jackie explained, "I trained on my own because I wanted to show everyone I could do it. I did ask people to train with me, but no one ever wanted to. However, once I began, I started meeting people who did the same thing I did. I met a few friends along the way that would go with me every once in awhile. The triathlon class was good too. I met some nice people with the same goals in mind.

"I also felt accountable to do these triathlons because I asked you to help me with them. I don't like to disappoint and especially not myself. When it comes down to it, I felt better doing it and I never had any regrets."

I asked how her weight was doing. "It stays the same," she frowned. "It bothers me because I'd like to lose five pounds for the next race." We started talking about eating and she didn't know how many calories she consumed on a daily basis, but told me her meals for that day: breakfast was a protein shake, snack was an apple or granola in yogurt, lunch was a turkey sandwich, and dinner would be steak and some leftover clam chowder. "I know the clam chowder isn't good for me," she said. I assured her it was okay in moderation. She then talked about eating peanuts after dinner. "I have a handful, maybe 10 or 20." I explained to her that if she were indeed trying to lose a few pounds, she would need to count out the peanuts to avoid mindless eating.

"I'm a social drinker," Jackie added. "If I go to someone's house and they ask if I want wine, I have it." Just like with the peanuts, I suggested she have one glass of wine instead of two. She said she planned to cut out wine for the next triathlon. The choice would be hers.

> *"There are no chips, cookies, sodas or junk food in our house...but there is wine!"*

We laughed. I like the fact that she doesn't have junk food in the house. Children will eat what's in the pantry and they can acquire a taste for unhealthy foods, things like fast food.

I asked if she felt ready for the Marsh Creek Triathlon in two months. "If I had to do it tomorrow, no — I have to keep up with all of it. I have to build back up." Then Jackie said, "I want to do this for years. I want to be in my 40s and still be doing races. Will or can I do it for years?" My answer was yes she could, because she was building a good foundation, listening to her body, cross training, eating well, and doing all the things she needed to do.

An added new benefit of Jackie's training was the increased interest her family was developing in exercise. Her 10-year-old son Nathan, who was a baseball and football player, but had not really run distance before, agreed to run a 5K with Jackie.

> *"Nathan was running a 5K after only a week of training," Jackie exclaimed. "It took me six months or so!"*

While training for the 5K, Nathan and Jackie ran in the rain one day and were drenched. "The only thing that stopped us," Jackie said, "was that my hairspray was running down into my eyes and I couldn't see. Running in the rain was fun though!"

Her 7-year-old daughter Kayla wanted to run too, but because she was smaller, she rode her scooter or bike. "It was fun to race her up the hill to see who could get there first," she laughed. Jackie smiled as she told me all this and it was heart-warming to see how pleased she was with her family's involvement.

We then had what I found to be a fascinating conversation about how she trains and how much she trains. Jackie explained to me how she trains just enough for each race and doesn't push herself beyond what she needs to do during the actual race. She noted, "I do the training just enough to be able to complete the race. That's how I do pretty much everything in my life, just enough to get by. Could I run more? Yes, but I don't.

"I know my potential is more but I also know I improve with each race. Other people tell me they left everything out there on the course but I don't feel the same way. I just know how it feels afterwards, when the race is over, and I love it!" This conversation reflected Jackie's personality and was one trait I hoped to explore later to find out why she feels "just enough" is okay.

After our get-together at the coffee shop Jackie was going to the YMCA to swim. My triathlon woman was addicted not only to all the different events she has to train for, but also to the feeling of finishing a workout and competing in a race.

An Unexpected Twist

Less than a week before the final race of the season — the much-anticipated Marsh Creek Triathlon — we were dealt a devastating blow. When Jackie went online to take a look at the previous year's results, she was shocked to see that she was not listed as a participant in the upcoming race. Now the race was full!

> *"I panicked and then pleaded with the race*
> *coordinator to see if I could get in, but to*
> *no avail," she said, "they had signed up 750*
> *competitors and were not taking any more."*

She had completed the online application process but hadn't received a confirmation number. Lesson learned.

Not only were Jackie's husband and children planning to wake up at 5:00 am on the morning of the race, I was going to surprise her by bringing my parents, who live nearby and had never seen a triathlon. They wanted to be there to cheer her on. The surprise would have been on us if we all showed up and were told Jackie couldn't race.

Jackie felt deflated! She wanted this race to complete the second year of training and competing. Now she scrambled to find a replacement race, and was even considering an upcoming triathlon that included an ocean swim. "Do you think I could do it?" Jackie asked. She had practiced an ocean swim earlier in the year in the warm waters of Florida and was able to complete a quarter-mile swim. But she struggled getting back out of the ocean with the waves crashing around her and pulling her back in.

The bigger concern, I explained to her was that this race would be in October, the water would be freezing and wetsuits would likely be mandatory. Jackie had never trained with a wetsuit and would need time getting used to it and being able to get out of a wetsuit quickly during T1.

Jackie admitted this would be a better goal to work toward next year and not something she should rush into. She was frantic and frazzled as she continued to find a replacement race. Her scheduling mistake had really disappointed her and she was afraid she had really let me down too. I have to admit it was an unexpected and frustrating turn of events.

Jackie found a triathlon for September 27th — or so she thought — where the swim would be in a pool. The bike course looked like a challenging one, which pleased Jackie because she trained on hills and really enjoyed them. I found this so funny coming from my once non-biker. When she sent me the information on the race I pointed out the date was actually the 26th.

"There must be something wrong with me," Jackie exclaimed. "I can't seem to get any of the details right lately!" Clearly she was frustrated and I asked if she was doing too much and should she slow down a bit. She admitted that she probably was moving in too many directions now. She worked at a fitness club each morning, still sold real estate, had her kitchenware business, the kids in school with homework, activities, household responsibilities, and her triathlon training on top of it all. "Yes it's a lot," she told me and added, "but it'll be okay.

> *"The one thing that keeps me in check, believe it or not, is my own fitness training. I would be even crazier without it!"*

To me it seemed like Jackie was doing too much, so I explained how I pick three things and focus on them. Doing this allows me to be the best I can at those three things, and I don't spread myself too thin. My three areas of focus are:

1. Being a personal trainer
2. Teaching fitness classes
3. Spreading the word about health and fitness through my books and presentations

Maybe this would work for her too. She agreed to think about it.

I awoke with a little sadness in my heart on the day that would have been Jackie's final triathlon — the final one to compare to last year. It was a crisp morning and I thought of how cold the water might have been in the lake. The sun was shining and they were calling for a gorgeous day, cool in the morning, no humidity, and then a sunny 75 degrees. It would have been ideal for a triathlon!

I wonder how Jackie would have done. Such a valuable lesson was learned. Always get a confirmation number or whatever necessary to confirm you have truly entered a race. I just can't imagine Jackie, her kids, her husband, my parents, and me all being there the morning of the race and Jackie being told she hadn't even entered.

I was upset at first, really frustrated, because I wanted to see how Jackie would do with this race. I wanted to be there. I wanted the race to be the final chapter of this book. I wanted us to be able to describe how well Jackie had competed. We could have told how she had learned so much over the past two years and how it had all come together for this final race. But, this isn't about me at all — it's Jackie's story.

Life does not always go as planned. I firmly believe things happen for a reason. Jackie was meant to have this shock, and quite a shock it was. I can almost guarantee this will never happen to her again. She will get a confirmation number or letter or whatever she needs in the future. Anyone reading this book will hopefully learn from Jackie's mistake. It was Jackie's sixth race and it happened to her; it could happen to anyone.

You ARE A Triathlete!

When Jackie awoke the morning of September 26th she was met with an unexpected sensation — a sense of calm. She was competing in her final triathlon of the year, one she had never done before, and yet she was not nervous. "I just felt good," she explained.

> *"I was able to compete in this triathlon as if*
> *I have been doing them my whole life. I was*
> *comfortable. The fear just left me as if I were*
> *setting out for a long walk in the park."*

Jackie was up at 5:00 am to leave for the hour and 15-minute drive. Todd was out of town so she was on her own for this race. Her sister stayed with the kids. The drive there was easy and Jackie actually enjoyed some time to herself.

The swim was at a YMCA pool. When Jackie arrived, she stood in line with at least 200 other participants. The swimmers had to count their own laps, which concerned her. "My only worry was losing count, my mind wanders off while I swim. I was told this was going to happen eventually," Jackie told me, "my mind would wander off and swimming would feel more natural." But she was able to focus and keep count and was soon outside on her bike in the crisp air. She started going in the wrong direction, but quickly corrected her course. Jackie was pleased to be one of the first 20 competitors to transition to the bike.

As they began the bike, Jackie and another woman kept passing each other and it appeared they would probably do so the whole way — but they didn't. In typical Jackie style, she took advantage of her love of downhill speed and the other woman was left behind. Jackie's next goal was to find another person to pass, which was a challenge to keep moving along. It was a difficult course, but Jackie's enjoyment of hills gave her an advantage. Her bike however locked up on her halfway up a steep hill and she had to get off, push it to a driveway, and fix it. She then had to get back on and start off midway up the hill. She was still calm and enjoyed the ride.

She passed a couple other people, but was pretty much alone the whole ride until she was passed by a couple of riders toward the end.

> *"What I find funny is that a lot of people are so nice to you when they pass you," Jackie smiled. "They have a mini-conversation with you as they pass as if to say 'sorry about that.' It's funny because even though it's a competition, once you are out there you feel like you're competing as part of a team of friends who are actually strangers!"*

Jackie finished the bike and started her run. She jogged; pacing herself as she knew the course would be hilly. A few of the hills brought on a slight charley horse so she had to finish walking up the hill to let it wear off. Much to her surprise, the woman she passed on her bike at the beginning was suddenly beside her again. She had caught up with Jackie and they ran the rest of the way together.

When Jackie felt like walking, the woman told Jackie to keep on running. She motivated Jackie to keep moving! They both crossed the finish line and the woman thanked Jackie for not passing her on the run like she had on the bike. Jackie thanked the woman for keeping her motivated and pushing her to not stop running. The camaraderie was incredible!

And that was it. The race was over. No big ending, but Jackie realized it was her big ending. She reflected on the past two years of training and races and said,

> *"I can now swim. I ride a bike and I run! Who would have ever thought? Certainly not me. Next year, there will be more triathlons and*

*I'll keep doing them and you never know. . .an
ocean swim may be in the future. I don't have
my stats from this race, but this time I am just
happy. I'm happy because I did something I
never thought I was capable of, and all that
matters to me now is how I feel about myself.
I always needed someone to pat me on the
back for something like this, but I feel amazing
because I did this for me."*

Jackie was not meant to do the second Marsh Creek Triathlon.
She was meant to do this one. She was meant to meet this woman.
Jackie had the courage and confidence to do it alone and not be
nervous.

Her reaction to this race made me feel this was the best ending
possible to Jackie's journey to a triathlon. It was race number six.
It astonishes me how, if you want, you can change your life. Jackie
is living proof that it can be done.

Who knew this "I can't swim. I don't own a bike and I hate to
run!" woman would turn out to be such an athlete?

Jackie, may you have many more years of triathlons. The world is
yours and you now realize that you can do anything you set your
mind to. I can't wait to hear what you want to do next.

You are a triathlete!

by Jackie Stenta

Growing up, exercise for me was playing outside with my sisters, throwing the ball around with my dad, or riding my bike to meet my friend. I thought of this as play and never considered it exercise. In high school, I could not even make it around the track without feeling faint. My first experience with exercise was right after my son Nathan was born. I joined a gym and started using the equipment. Then, after my daughter Kayla was born it really hit me. I needed to work out! I hired a trainer and exercise became a part of my life.

A few years went by and exercise started to feel more like work. I was uninspired to get up early to go to the gym or even work out at home. I was bored. Then something happened I never saw coming. Linda came into my life. She suggested a triathlon as a way to work towards a goal and feel a sense of accomplishment. We made an appointment and the rest, as they say, is history — or at least it's the story you just read.

When I look back over the past two years of training and competing, I see how much I have changed. I am not only stronger physically, but mentally as well. I learned that I do not want to have any regrets and if there were no tomorrow, I would want to feel proud of what I had accomplished and not say "what if" or "if only." My life is my own and it is up to me to make the best of it. There are no excuses; I am 100 percent accountable for how I feel and for what I will become.

Two years ago I was simply taking exercise classes, now I work at a gym leading classes and helping others achieve their goals.

I would never have had that confidence before. My kids now run with me, bike with me, and do workout videos with me. Exercise is a wonderful part of me that I can share with my family and help my children develop an appreciation for a healthy lifestyle.

I now get up between 5:00 and 6:00 am to work out. Believe me I still love my sleep, that hasn't changed, I just go to bed a little earlier. People ask me all the time why I am crazy enough to get up and go to the gym at that time of day, and my answer is always the same, "it stinks when I have to get up, but the feeling I get after it's over is so worth it."

Getting up early to go to the gym can be a challenge for me. I also think we sometimes view people in our lives as obstacles. They are easy targets to blame when we feel like we cannot do something. I realize now that it wasn't Todd who lacked confidence in my abilities; it was me.

Before, I would never work out in front of him because I thought he would tease me. Todd's cautious way of thinking may make his remarks sound negative, but his actions are always supportive — he cleans the house, never complains when I leave to train for my triathlons and he has the kids, etc. When it comes right down to it, he's my biggest supporter.

Now we work out together. He even bought me a bike to do triathlons! I could have easily assumed that a bike was too expensive and that my husband would never go for it, and not have asked. I told Todd about the triathlons and just like that, I had a bike. I should have asked for a spa vacation instead, right?

Triathlons scared me at first, especially the swimming. Recently I was at the pool talking to the lifeguards. We laughed about the times when I first started learning how to swim and would go to the pool. I would stand at the wall, take a deep breath, and get ready to get my head in the water and then stop.

I would hesitate to put my head in the water for the first 15 minutes and would keep starting and stopping, just standing in the pool. It must have been a funny sight! The lifeguards would come and ask if I was okay and I would tell them I was just warming up. And there was the swimming in lakes and ponds. I never wanted to get into a lake with live creatures! Never, never, never! But I did.

Then came the running — I hated it! No, I actually despised it. I hated to have to breathe that hard. Todd would go running and then come back and tell me I should try. I would say "That will be the day! You'll never see me run. I hate running."

Linda taught me all about taking baby steps. Start out slowly, one step at a time. It was like feeding children vegetables, they may not like them at first, but little by little over time, they will start to want more.

There was a time during this training I questioned why I could not push myself to do more while I was out at the triathlon. I think I answered my question on why that is.

At my final triathlon, when I finished I felt calm. I did not feel overly exhausted or weak. I felt strong and I also felt I could have kept going. I think that was an important wall to break through in training for triathlons. I thought I WAS pushing myself and all the while I think in my head I always felt I could do better. But sometimes your body can only do so much. So my brain and my body were thinking two different things. My brain was saying, "I know you can kick it up a notch" and my body was saying "Are you crazy? Just keep pacing yourself."

At my final triathlon I finally broke past that and I pushed myself up another level. Every time I do a race I beat my previous time. So instead of beating myself up thinking I could do better, all the while I WAS doing better. I just had to start somewhere.

The best part of doing triathlons was seeing the look on my family's face when I finished each race. The reason I know I can keep moving forward is that I have a great support system. You need internal drive to start a race, but often it's the external support you get that pushes you to finish. Sometimes we don't even realize what a great support system we have when we start out.

Have you ever started something new and tell your family and friends about it, only to hear all the negative reasons why you shouldn't do it? They think they are helping you and protecting you because they only want what's best for you. It was this fear that kept me from originally telling anyone about my intentions.

When I started training for triathlons, I did not tell the people closest to me. I wanted to see what I could do first. When I did tell them, they were proud of me and offered their unconditional support. I was especially worried about how Todd would react.

What I have learned about my husband through this experience is that although he initially pointed out the negatives, in the end he became my biggest supporter. He now drives me to triathlons, helps me with my bags and bike, and has bought me sneakers, sport watches, a bike, and triathlon clothes.

I know I will keep doing triathlons. I want to see where this will take me. My goal is to stick to three triathlons per year and each year add another piece of gear to help me improve my race. I would also like to add an ocean swim in the next year or two, which will depend on how often I can make it to the ocean to practice. I just need enough time to go to learn how to get into the ocean and then get back out. Once I am in I know I can do it.

Triathlons are part of my life. I don't think I could stop now. I like doing the races and I also like to swim! I like to run! I love to bike! See, I can at least say I like them. Biking ended up being my favorite! And for me to say that I even like the other two — that is far off from hating it before!

Every now and then I take time off. I have not been swimming in a few weeks, but that's okay. Sometimes you need time off to give yourself a break. I am looking forward to getting back in the pool next week, right back on the schedule again.

If you are considering training for a triathlon, my advice is to find it within yourself and go for it! Pick out the most supportive people in your life and let them help you achieve your goals. My parents always told me that I could do anything. When I talked to them, there was never any doubt in their minds that I could climb mountains if I chose to!

My husband, though very silent, is always standing by me when I need him. He is the reason I push myself to be better. When I compete in triathlons, I think of him and I move a little faster. My kids are my cheering squad and are always ready to receive a sweaty hug at the finish line making it all worthwhile! Linda has a way of making everything seem so easy. Her contagious personality and enthusiasm are inspirational!

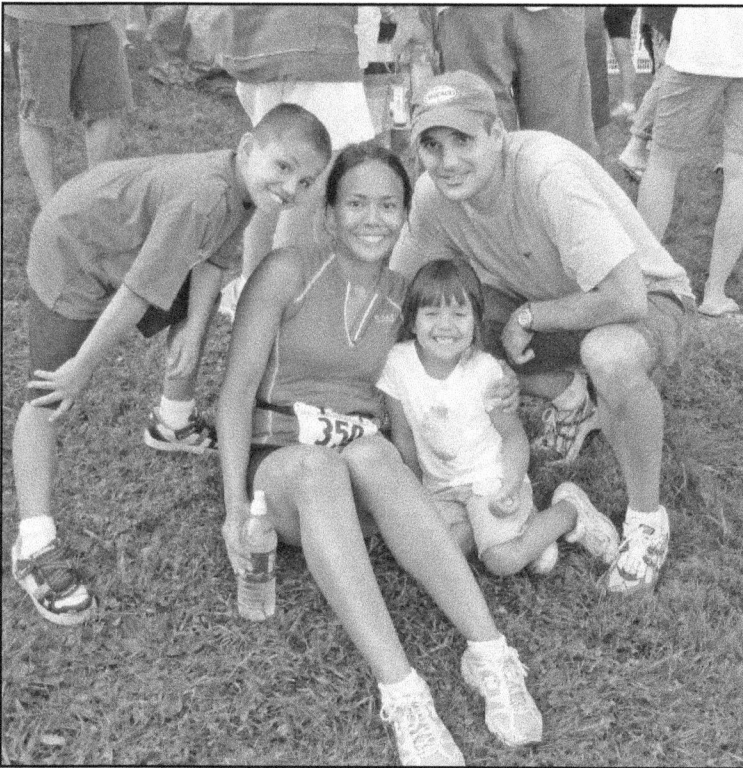

Nathan, Jackie, Kayla and Todd at the
Marsh Creek Triathlon

— Notes —

— Notes —

— Notes —

www.ingramcontent.com/pod-product-compliance
Lightning Source LLC
Chambersburg PA
CBHW070851280326
41934CB00008B/1396